Also he must know the Anatomie:- for those Surgeons that work in man's body not knowing Anatomie is likened to a blind man that cutteth a Vine Tree, for he taketh away more or lesse than he ought to doo

From *The Qualities of a Surgeon* Thomas Vicary (1490-1562)

# A Colour Atlas of Surgical Anatomy of the Abdomen in the Living Subject

**Roy Yorke Calne**

# A Colour Atlas of
# Surgical Anatomy
# of the Abdomen

## in the living subject

**Sir Roy Calne**
FRCS FRS
*Professor of Surgery, University of Cambridge*

With radiological contributions from
**Adrian K. Dixon**
MA MRCP FRCR
*Lecturer in Radiology, University of Cambridge*
*Honorary Consultant Radiologist, Addenbrooke's Hospital, Cambridge*
and
**Derek S. Appleton**
MA FRCR
*Consultant Radiologist, Addenbrooke's Hospital, Cambridge*

**Wolfe Medical Publications Limited**
**Year Book Medical Publishers, Inc.**

# Dedication

To my children
Jane, Sarah, Deborah, Suzanne, Russell and Richard

Copyright © R.Y.Calne, 1988
Published by Wolfe Medical Publications Limited, 1988
Printed by Toppan Printing Co. (S) Pte. Ltd., Singapore

UK ISBN 0 7234 0888 2
USA ISBN 0 8151 1464 8

This book is one of the titles in the series of Wolfe Medical Atlases, a series which brings together probably the world's largest systematic published collection of diagnostic colour photographs.
    For a full list of Atlases in the series, plus forthcoming titles and details of our surgical, dental and veterinary Atlases, please write to Wolfe Medical Publications Limited, 2-16 Torrington Place, London WC1E 7LT, England
*or*
Year Book Medical Publishers, Inc., 200 North LaSalle Street, Chicago, Illinois 60601, USA.

**Library of Congress Cataloging-in-Publication Data**

Calne, Roy Yorke.
    Surgical anatomy of the abdomen.

    Includes index.
    1. Abdomen—Anatomy—Atlases. 2. Abdomen—Surgery—Complications and sequelae—Atlases. 3. Anatomy, Surgical and topographical—Atlases. I. Title.
[DNLM: 1. Abdomen—anatomy & histology—atlases.
2. Abdomen—surgery—atlases. WI 17 C164s]
QM543.C35 1988    611'.95    87-29429
ISBN 0-8151-1464-8

*Distributed in Continental North America*
*Hawaii and Puerto Rico by*
Year Book Medical Publishers, Inc.

# Preface

Since the Renaissance work of Leonardo da Vinci and Vesalius, the cadaver has been the basis of both the learning and the teaching of anatomy. During the nineteenth and the first half of the twentieth centuries the details of topographical anatomy were described, painted, modelled and photographed. Medical students and surgeons in training were required to have a sound knowledge of the structure of the body, but the curriculum tended to be cluttered with unimportant minutiae often unrelated to surgery. In the last twenty years new biochemistry, molecular biology, neurophysiology, embryology and other less well defined subjects have over-burdened the medical student.

There has been a neglect of topographical anatomy that can leave the student at the time of qualification seriously handicapped without a grasp of the essential structure of the species he has elected to doctor. The clinical student attending his first surgical operation is surprised how different the perfused living tissues and organs are to the dead specimens and illustrations that he has superficially studied.

In this volume, I have considered anatomy from the point of view of the general surgeon and attempted to relate structure to function so that disturbances of structure in surgical diseases can explain symptoms, signs and deranged function. Some examples are given of the anatomical changes that can follow obstruction of hollow viscera. Photographs of living anatomy are supplemented by radiographs and simple illustrations. I have not written a formal, detailed text since there are many excellent descriptions of anatomy in print. It is hoped that this applied presentation will be easily understood and of interest to medical students, surgeons in training and theatre nurses.

# Acknowledgements

In preparing this book I am indebted to many colleagues for their generous help and I thank my daughter, Deborah, for many hours spent in compilation of text and illustrations and for the outlining of most of the diagrams and my secretary, Miss Audrey Campbell, for the typing of illegible manuscripts. Mr Michael Smith and many of the staff in Addenbrooke's who have helped take the photographs; the Medical Photography Department of Addenbrooke's, Mr Paul Smith and Mrs Geneva Moore have processed many of the films and Drs Vivian Lees and Richard Scott demonstrated the power of the abdominal muscles.

I am especially grateful to Dr Gordon Wright, Mr Simon Harrison, Mr Robert Greatorex and Professor M. Balasegaram for their suggestions relating to the script and I thank Mr Turner Warwick for his aid in explaining and illustrating the urinary sphincters and Dr Sathia Thiru for the histological figures and their legends. I thank my colleagues, Messrs Doyle, Dunn, Everett, Yadav, Friend, Elias-Jones, and Professor Thomas Sherwood for providing figures.

Lastly I am most grateful to my radiological colleagues, Drs Appleton and Dixon who contributed most of the radiographs, CT scans and their legends.

I was deeply saddened by the death of Mr Peter Wolfe during the gestation of this book. His enthusiasm and encouragement were of great help to me.

# Contents

# Introduction

This book is an attempt to help the medical student, junior surgical trainee and operating theatre nurse appreciate and understand the living anatomy of the abdomen, the chief work site of the general surgeon.

Since access and exposure is often limited, the surgeon uses fingers nearly as much as eyes in assessing anatomy. To do this he must be familiar with the texture, shape and relations of the abdominal organs.

All surgical procedures depend on healing and the single most important requirement for this is a good blood supply. Thus, although the anatomy of nerves and lymphatics may be key features in certain operations, the blood supply is essential in all cases.

Three recent technical developments have been used in this book that were not available to the great traditional anatomists of the past.

**A** Modern anaesthesia permits very extensive surgical dissections, so that unusual views of perfused organs can be obtained, for example, the hepatic fossa can be seen empty in the preparation of a recipient for a liver graft (**1**) and the whole opened abdomen can be displayed in a multi-organ donor, with brain stem death but an intact circulation (**2-6**).

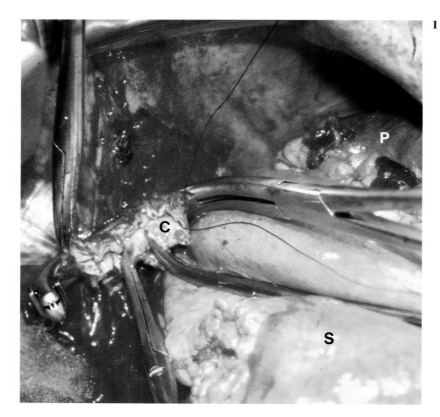

**1** Shows the empty hepatic fossa, the liver having been removed. There is a clamp on the diaphragm containing the cut vena cava (C). Stomach (S) and spleen (P) can be seen.

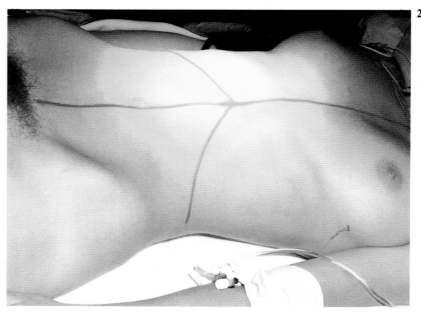

**2** The incision for removal of organs in a case of brain stem and cerebral destruction. With the circulation intact, the heart, liver, kidneys and pancreas can be removed for transplantation.

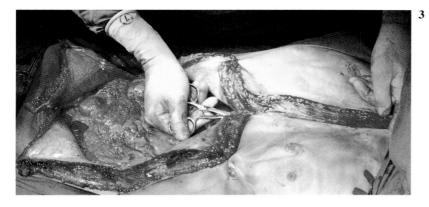

**3** The abdominal incision has been made, the abdomen opened and the forceps have been passed behind the sternum, in front of the pericardium to allow a Gigli saw to be used to open and divide the sternum longitudinally.

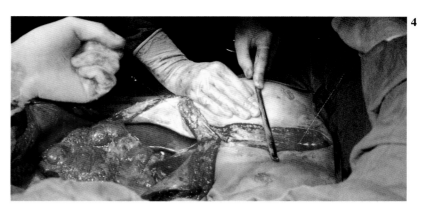

**4** Shows the saw in action.

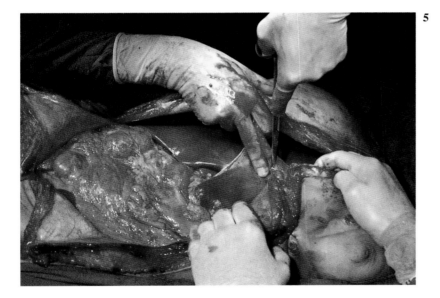

**5** The sternum has been split. The falciform ligament has been divided. The liver can be seen in the middle.

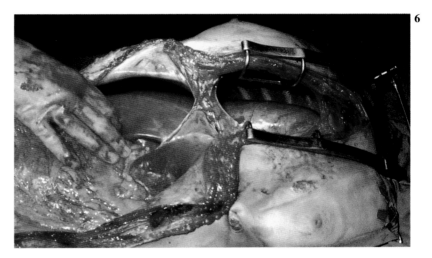

**6** A self-retaining retractor has been inserted to facilitate exposure.

**B**  High resolution film emulsion and flash permit rapid close-up photography with good depth of focus. The photographer does not require elaborate preparation with a tripod and special lighting. He can pop over the surgeon's shoulder, and at the appropriate moment, with a hand held camera, press the shutter release and quickly retire.

**C**  Computed tomography and angiography demonstrate anatomy in the intact patient, showing the relations and vascularisation of tissues and organs, which can then be seen directly at surgery (**7-25**).

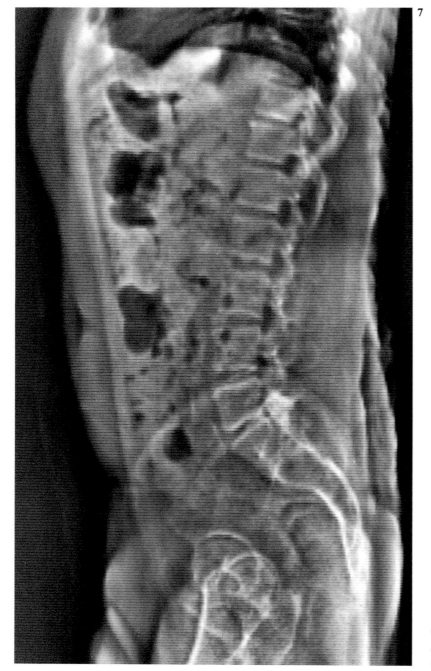

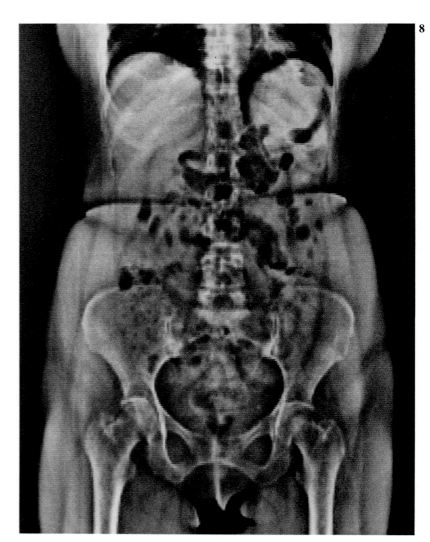

**8**  An anteroposterior view of the abdomen showing the rib cage, spine and pelvis.

**7**  A longitudinal digital radiograph of the abdomen showing the lumbar spine curving convexly anteriorly. Sacrum below and the rib cage above. Pelvis and femoral heads and necks can be seen.

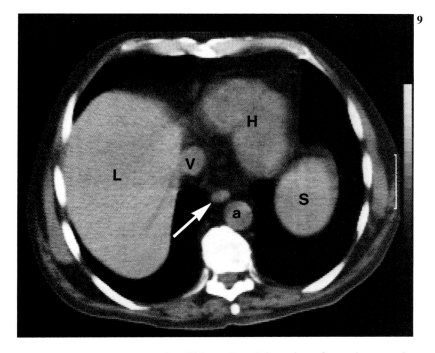

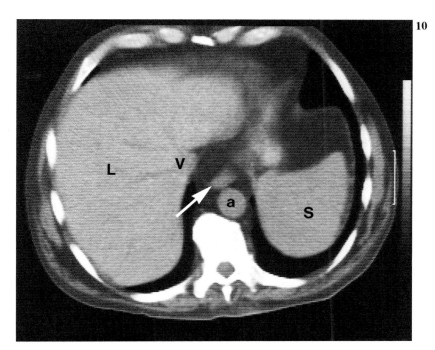

**9-23** Computed tomography (CT scan) serial sections from above at the junction of the chest and abdomen to below the caudal extremity of the sacrum. In each photograph the vertebral column is in the midline posteriorly. Organs are viewed as if looked at from below. The organs on the patient's right appear on the left hand side of the picture and vice versa.

**9,10** Aorta (a), heart (H), oesophagus (arrow), vena cava (V), liver (L), spleen (S), and lower thoracic cage can be seen.

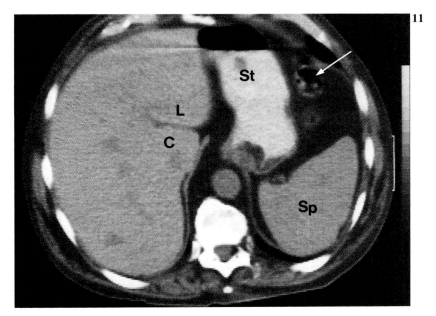

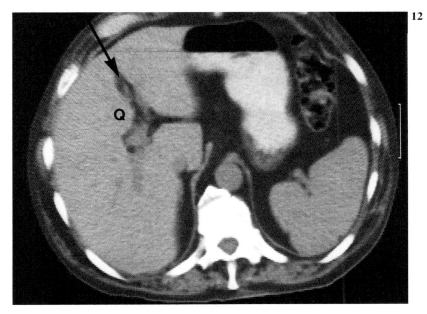

**11** The tip of the splenic flexure of the colon can be seen anteriorly on the left (arrow). Air/fluid level within stomach (St). The fissure of the lesser omentum can be seen between the posterior aspect of the left lobe (L) and caudate (C) lobes of liver. Spleen (Sp).

**12** The falciform ligament (arrow) can be seen between the lateral segment and the medial segment of the left lobe of the liver with its quadrate surface (Q) posteriorly. Just behind the quadrate surface the portal vein can be seen in the porta hepatis.

13

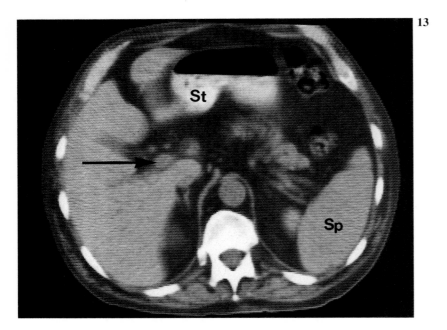

**13**  The next cut shows the portal vein (arrowed) just anterior to the caudate lobe of the liver. The normal hepatic artery and common bile duct can be seen just anterior to the portal vein. The distal body and tail of the pancreas can be seen anterior to the vessels supplying the spleen (Sp). Note the air in the anterior portion of the body of the stomach (St) which runs transversely from left to right at this level.

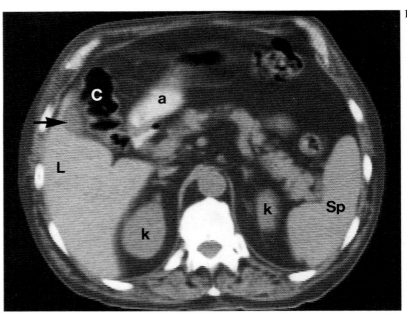

**14**  The upper poles of both kidneys (k) are now well seen. The pancreatic tail is shown extending to the hilum of the spleen (Sp). The hepatic flexure of the colon (C) is anterior to the gall bladder (arrow) which in turn is anterior to the right lobe of the liver (L). The antrum (a) of the stomach is now directed posteriorly.

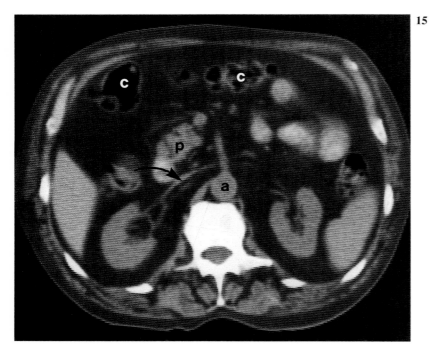

**15**  The superior mesenteric artery takes its origin from the anterior aspect of the aorta (a). The inferior vena cava (arrowed) is slit-like on this cut; both renal veins can be seen entering it. A small portion of the right renal artery can be seen just posterior to the cava. The head and uncinate process of pancreas (p) are lateral to the superior mesenteric vessels. The transverse colon (c) can be seen anteriorly.

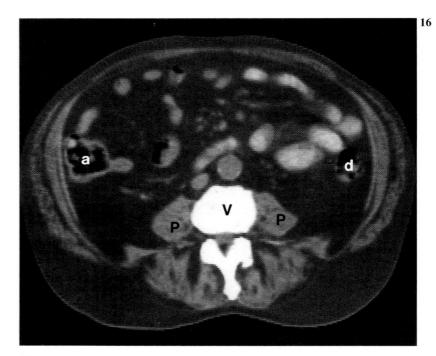

**16**  Below the kidneys, both psoas muscles (P) are on either side of the L4 vertebral body (V). The ascending (a) and descending (d) portions of the colon are well seen in the retroperitoneal fat.

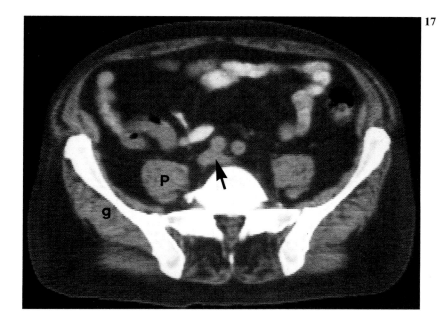

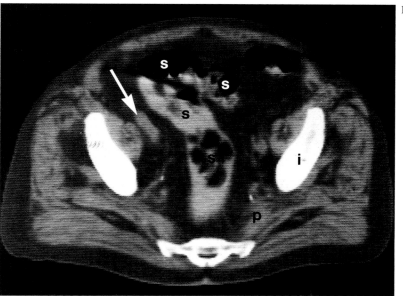

**17** The aorta has now bifurcated and both common iliac arteries are seen anterior to the confluence of the two iliac veins (arrowed) anterior to the 1st sacral vertebra. The three layers of the anterior abdominal wall musculature are clearly defined laterally. The gluteal muscles (g) can be seen posterolateral to the iliac wings. The psoas muscles (P) are again shown.

**18** The anterior position and tortuosity of the sigmoid colon (s) can be well appreciated as it passes posteriorly from the false pelvis towards the rectum within the true pelvis. The piriformis muscle (p) can be seen passing through the greater sciatic notch between sacrum and iliac bone (i). The external iliac vessels (arrow) are just anteromedial to the iliopsoas.

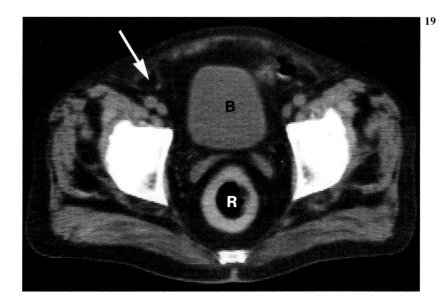

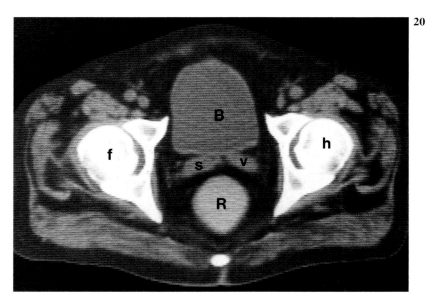

**19** An image obtained through the acetabular roofs. The internal ring (arrow) of the right inguinal canal can be seen anterior to the external iliac vessels; at this point the external iliac artery passes under the inguinal ligament to become the femoral artery. Between the bladder (B) and the rectum (R), the cranial portions of both seminal vesicles can be seen.

**20** At the level of the femoral heads (f, h) within the acetabular cups. The seminal vesicles (s, v) are closely applied to the posterior aspect of the bladder (B) and closely related to the anterior wall of the rectum (R). The coccyx is posterior to the rectum.

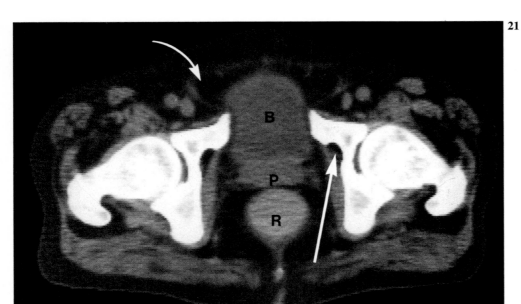

**21** The femoral heads and necks are well seen. The obturator foramen (straight arrow) is seen just lateral to the obturator internus muscle. Both inguinal canals (curved arrow) are anteromedial to the femoral vessels. The relationships of the bladder (B), prostate (P) and rectum (R) can be well appreciated.

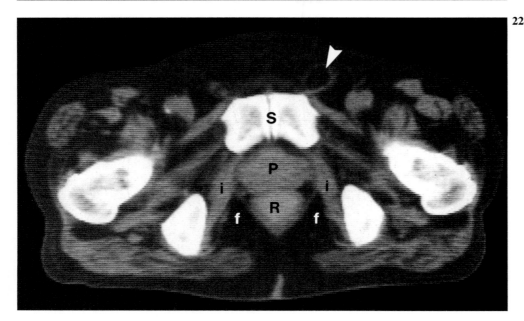

**22** At the level of the pubic symphysis (S). The external ring (arrow) of the left inguinal canal is seen attached to the pubic tubercle. The prostate (P) is anterior to the distal rectum (R). The thin levator ani muscles can just be seen on either side of the rectum. They form the anteromedial wall of the ischio-rectal fossae (f). The internal obturator muscles (i) form the anterolateral walls.

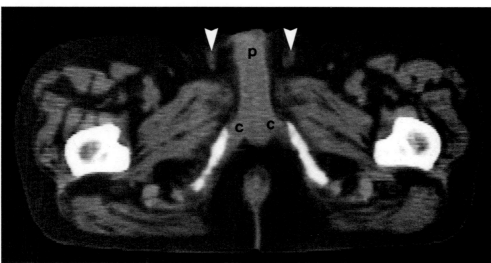

**23** Cut through inferior pubic rami and caudal aspect of ischial bones. Both ischiocavernosus muscles (c) can be seen contributing to the penis (p). Both spermatic cords can also be seen (arrows).

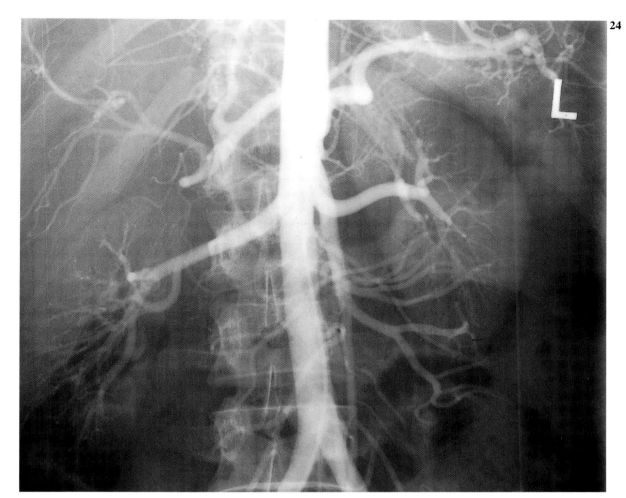

**24** Flush aortogram – arterial phase. X-ray was taken after a catheter had been inserted into the right femoral artery and passed up into the upper abdominal aorta. The aorta and bifurcation are outlined, the bifurcation opposite the body of L4

From above downwards the following can be seen: the coeliac axis and its branches with the hepatic artery on the right and splenic on the left; the superior mesenteric artery passing to the left of the aorta longitudinally downwards, giving off branches to the small bowel; the two main renal arteries.

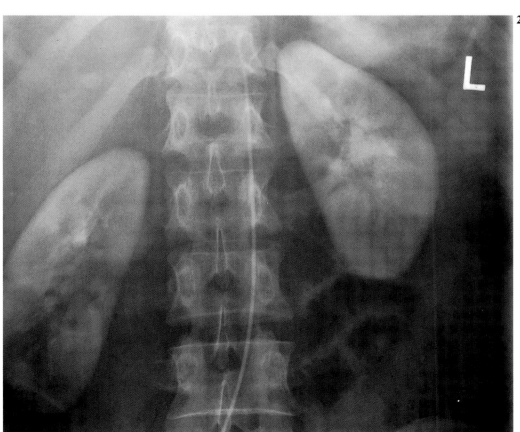

**25** Flush aortogram – venous phase. Both kidneys are now clearly seen with renal veins passing medially. The spleen is outlined above the left kidney and the portal vein is seen over the liver.

# 1 General Description of the Abdomen and its Contents – *Laparotomy*

The abdomen is beautifully designed to accommodate the organs it contains and fulfil their various requirements. It is a muscular, expansile case with a semi-rigid supporting spine. Throughout life the dome-shaped, muscular and tendinous *diaphragm* that separates the abdominal from the thoracic cavity, descends by contraction of its muscle fibres to increase the size of the chest and cause lung expansion. It then relaxes during expiration. The descent of the diaphragm varies in extent and interval – slow and regular in sleep, greatest and fastest during exercise.

When the diaphragm descends, the organs directly abutting it are also pushed downwards. This can be demonstrated by palpation and percussion of the liver, spleen and kidneys, especially when they are enlarged. The stomach, due to its hollow structure and soft walls, moves less with respiration, but a rigid stomach infiltrated with growth may move with the diaphragm. The muscular, abdominal wall relaxes during inspiration. Contraction of the abdominal wall muscles helps to fix the spine so that the trunk can form a supporting plinth for the arms and legs to make forceful movements. The tight abdominal wall of an athlete holds the intra-abdominal organs firmly in place (**26, 27**) yet in pregnancy the abdominal muscles can relax and allow the uterus to fill the expanded abdominal cavity to accommodate a 5 kg foetus (**28**).

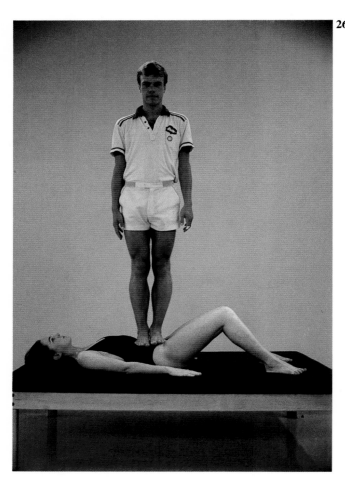

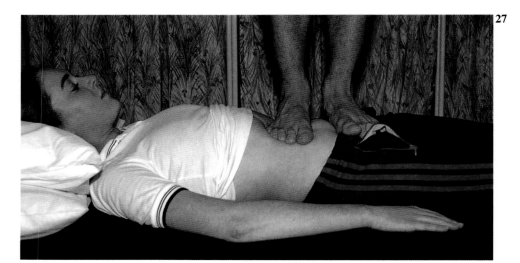

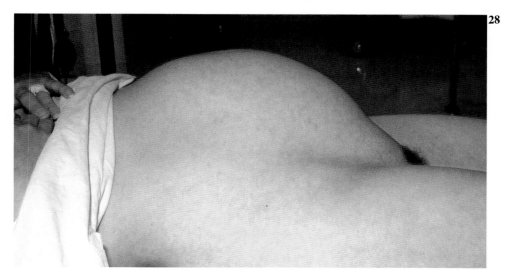

**26,27** The abdominal muscles of a trained athlete are remarkably strong, as shown in these pictures where the full weight of a man is held comfortably by the anterior abdominal wall of a young woman who is a black belt in karate.

**28** Shows the ability of the abdominal wall muscles to relax physiologically in advanced pregnancy.

The *bony pelvis* is shaped like a basin, open at both ends (**29**). The wide orifice of the false pelvis is in continuity with the main abdominal cavity. The narrow true pelvis contains the bladder, rectum and female reproductive tract. The female pelvis is wider and tapers less than the male to permit passage of the foetus during birth. The subpubic angle and greater sciatic notches are 90° or more, whilst in the male both these form acute angles. The male pelvic bones are thicker and the acetabula are relatively larger than those of the female pelvis (**30, 31**). The pelvis has a complicated system of muscles that control the exits of the urinary, gastro-intestinal and female reproductive tracts.

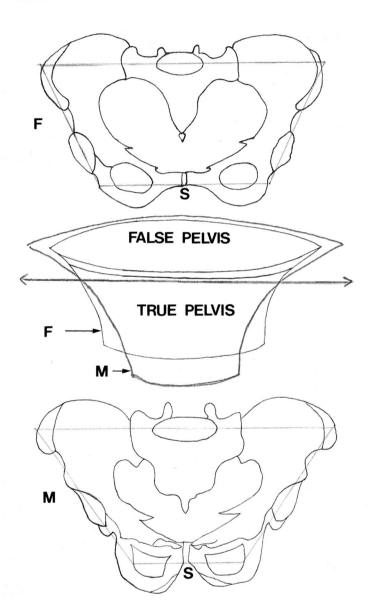

**29** Diagram of the female pelvis (F) above and male pelvis (M) below showing the resemblance of the pelvis to a basin, the upper part being the false pelvis and the lower part the true pelvis. Subpubic angle (S).

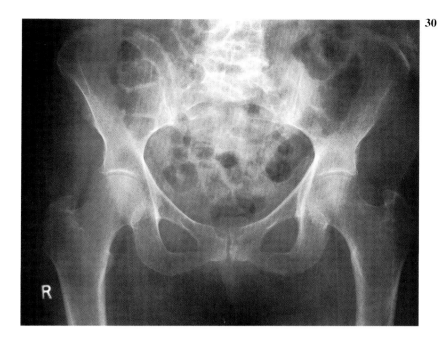

**30** X-ray of the female pelvis.

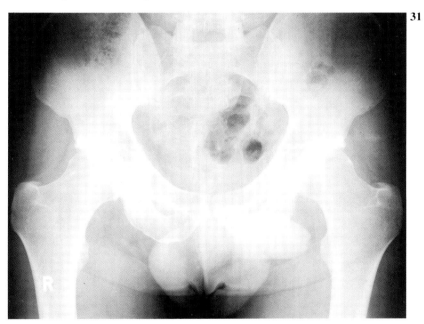

**31** X-ray of the male pelvis.

The *lumbar spine* is curved convex forwards (lordosis) and divides the posterior wall of the abdomen into right and left compartments (**7-17**). In front of the lumbar vertebral bodies on each side lies the *lumbar sympathetic nerve chain* connecting the *lumbar ganglia*. The *aorta* runs on the left and the inferior vena cava on the right of the midline in front of the lumbar vertebral bodies. The large, powerful *psoas muscles* lie on each side of the lumbar spine between the vertebral bodies and their transverse processes. The *lumbar nerve plexus* is formed within the psoas muscle and the *sacral plexus* is formed in front of the *piriformis* muscle in the pelvis. These two important nerve plexuses supply the lower limbs.

Anterior to the psoas muscles are the kidneys and ureters, above the kidneys lie the adrenal glands (**32**). The head of the pancreas is on the right of the body of L1, the body and neck of the pancreas cross the spine and the tail lies close to the spleen (**33**). The irregular shaped liver fills the right hypochondrium. The spleen and stomach occupy the left hypochondrium (**34**). The small bowel lies in the centre of the abdominal cavity (**35**). The large bowel courses around the periphery from the right iliac fossa in front of the right kidney, under the right lobe of the liver and across the abdomen to just below the spleen, descending in front of the left kidney to the pelvis.

This very brief summary forms the basis of the general exploratory laparotomy that a surgeon should undertake every time he opens the abdomen.

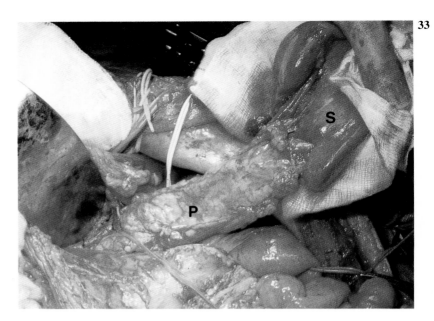

**33**

**33**  Shows the relationship of the tail of the pancreas (P) and the hilum of the spleen (S), in this case the pancreas and spleen have been mobilised from their normal position and are still attached to each other.

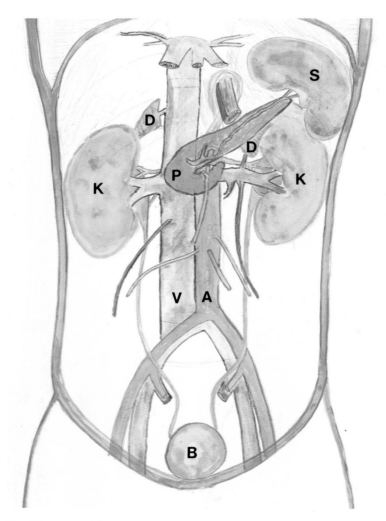

**32**

**32**  Diagram of the retroperitoneal organs, showing the relationship of the aorta (A) and vena cava (V) to the kidneys (K), adrenals (D), pancreas (P), bladder (B) and spleen (S).

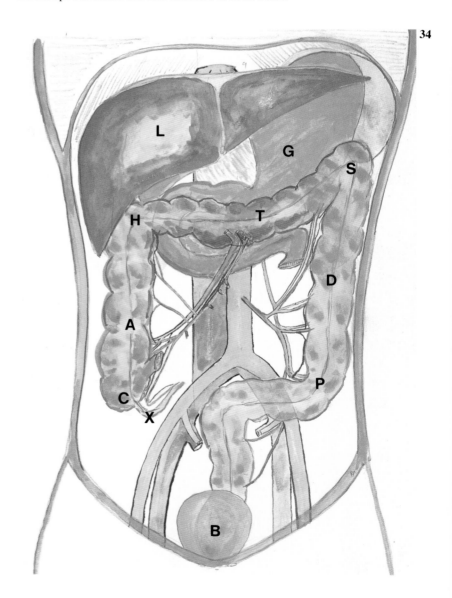

**34**

**34**  Diagram of the topography of the main abdominal organs. Liver (L), ascending colon (A), hepatic flexure (H), transverse colon (T), splenic flexure (S), descending colon (D), pelvic colon (P), bladder (B), caecum (C), appendix (X) and stomach (G).

# Laparotomy

A midline incision is made, extending from 6 cm above to 6 cm below the umbilicus, through the *linea alba*, a dense collagen band formed by interlacing of the aponeuroses of the muscles of both sides of the anterior abdominal wall. It stretches from the xiphoid process to the pubic symphysis. The parietal peritoneal lining of the abdominal cavity is then opened revealing its glistening inner face (36). It is reflected over the surface of the intra-abdominal organs as visceral peritoneum. The peritoneum reaches the mobile organs by double folds called *mesenteries* within which lie the blood and lymphatic vessels, lymph nodes and nerves (37, 38). The mesothelial peritoneal cells secrete peritoneal fluid which acts as a lubricant so that the mobile intra-abdominal organs can move freely without friction.

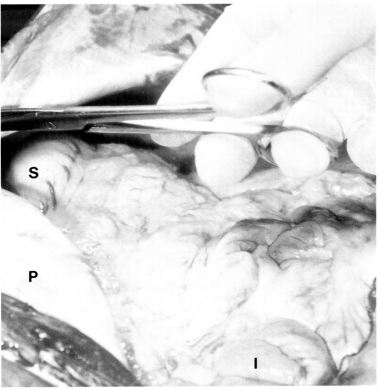

**36**

**36** Horizontal abdominal incision with midline upper extension. The upper flaps have been folded backwards showing the glistening parietal peritoneum (P). The stomach (S) to the left, and the intestines (I) lower right, are covered with visceral peritoneum.

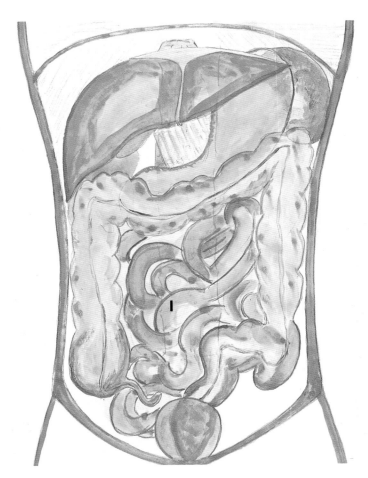

**35**

**35** Diagram of the abdominal contents, the anterior abdominal wall removed. The distribution of the small bowel (I) and its relation to the colon are shown.

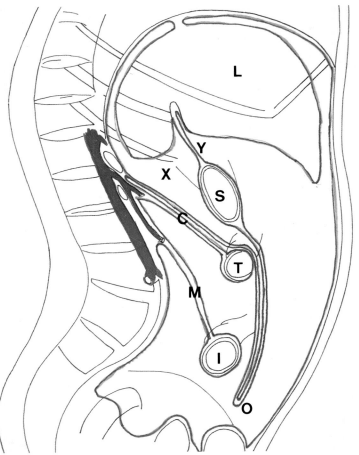

**37**

**37** Diagram of the sagittal section of the abdomen showing the parietal and visceral peritoneum and the omentum. Liver (L), stomach (S), transverse colon (T), small intestine (I), greater omentum (O), lesser omentum (Y), lesser sac (X), mesocolon (C), mesentery (M).

The first structures encountered within the abdominal cavity are the stomach and the *greater omentum* (**39, 40**). This greater omentum is an apron-like structure of peritoneum which hangs down from the greater curvature of the stomach in two layers, which pass over the transverse colon down into the lower abdomen. They then double back underneath the anterior layers, to which they fuse. The posterior layers continue upwards to enclose the transverse colon and become continuous with the transverse mesocolon. The greater omentum contains blood and lymphatic vessels and a variable amount of fat. It has a tendency to stick to areas of inflammation, walling them off and preventing spread of infection. It has been called the 'abdominal policeman'. It may be utilised surgically for the same purpose (**41, 42**). Standing on the patient's right, the right hand of the surgeon is passed upwards along the surface of the omentum.

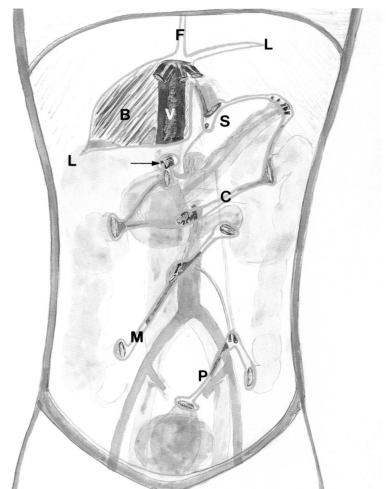

**38**

**38** Diagram of the posterior aspect of the peritoneal cavity showing the origins of the mesenteries and the peritoneal attachments of the liver. Falciform ligament (F), triangular ligaments (L), diaphragm in contact with bare area (B), inferior vena cava (V), free edge of lesser omentum (arrow), lesser sac (S), origin of transverse mesocolon (C), origin of mesentery (M), origin of pelvic mesocolon (P).

**39** Shows the abdominal contents after a transverse incision, revealing the edge of the liver uppermost (L), then the bulging stomach (S) and the omentum (O) which has been taken out of the wound.

**40** The omentum has been lifted up to show the lattice-work of blood vessels in the quadruple layers of peritoneum which contain fat in variable amounts.

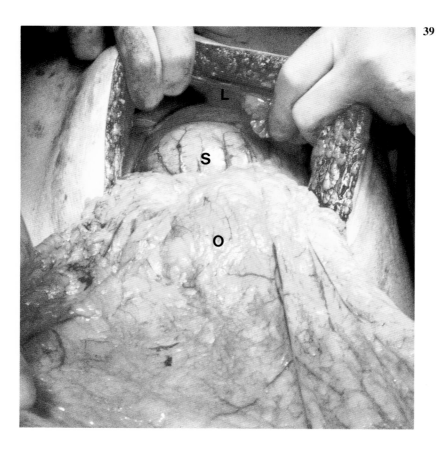

**39**

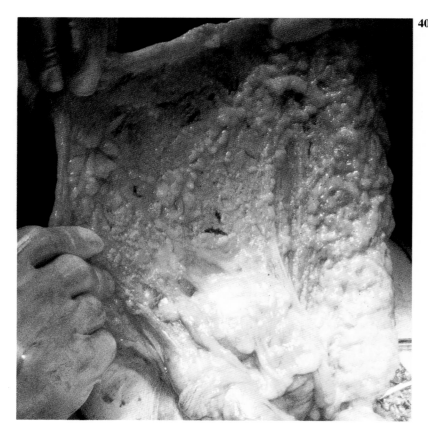

**40**

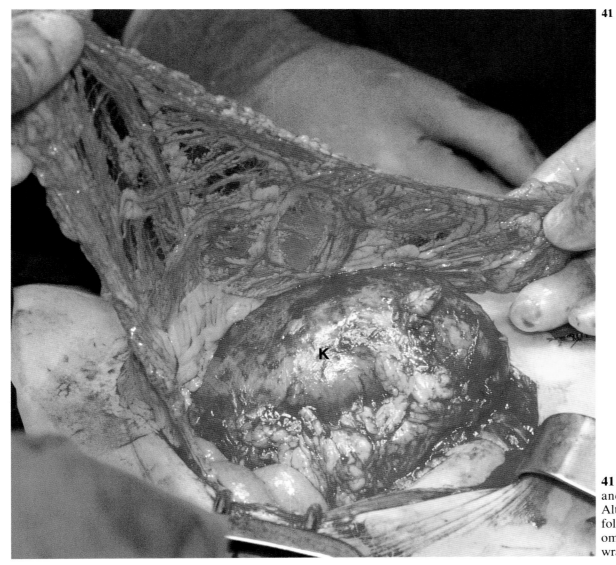

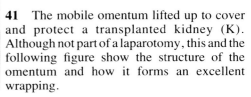

**41** The mobile omentum lifted up to cover and protect a transplanted kidney (K). Although not part of a laparotomy, this and the following figure show the structure of the omentum and how it forms an excellent wrapping.

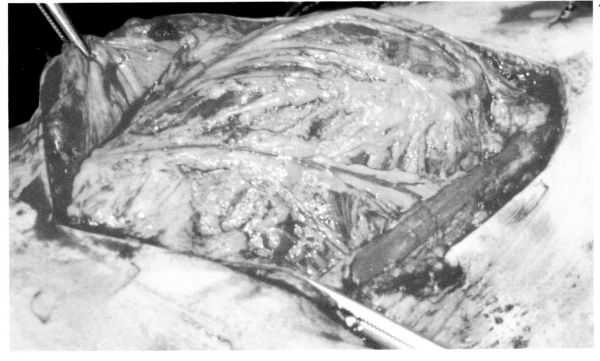

**42** The omentum loosely wrapped over the kidney to protect it.

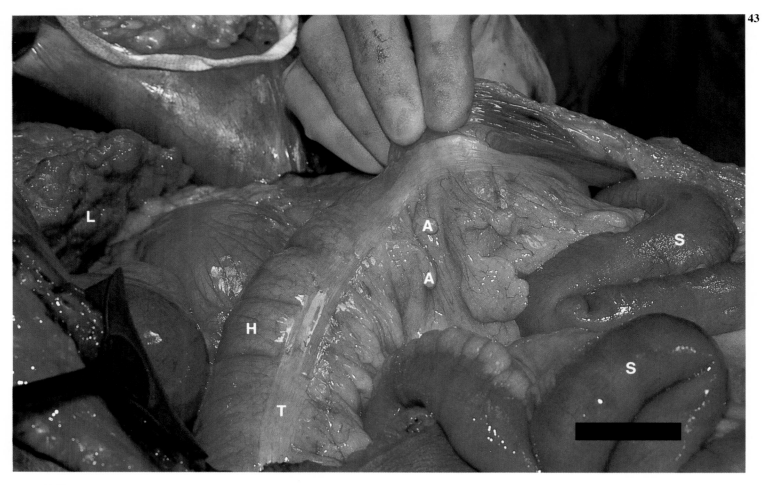

**43** Shows the transverse colon with longitudinal band, one of the three taenia in the middle (T). The little fatty appendices epiploicae (A) can be seen and on the convex border the haustrations (H) are easily identified as the sac-like bulges of the bowel between horizontal indentations which do not go the full width of the bowel. The small intestine (S) lies in coils to the right. The liver (L) is shrunken and nodular due to advanced cirrhosis.

If the greater omentum is lifted up the transverse colon will be seen, pinkish-grey in colour and soft in consistency with three longitudinal band-like structures of smooth muscle – the *taeniae coli* – on the surface (**43**). The colon has transverse indentations between which are sac like bulges called *haustrations* (**44**) and little fatty *appendices epiploicae* are dotted on the surface of the bowel where blood vessels enter the wall. The transverse colon can be lifted up and with the omentum elevated, the transverse mesocolon, containing the *middle colic vessels* can be seen. There may be indentible and moveable faeces in the lumen of the bowel.

**44**

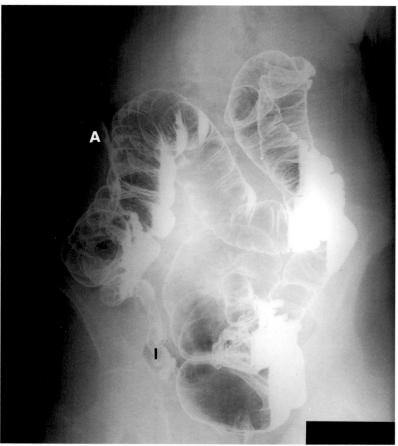

**44** Double contrast barium enema (showing fluid levels), with the patient lying in the left decubitus position. The characteristic configuration of the large bowel with haustrations, can be seen. Note also some reflux into normal terminal ileum (I) and a long retrocaecal appendix (A).

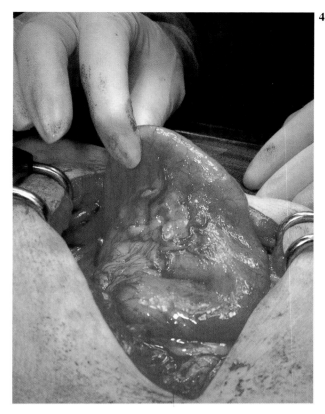

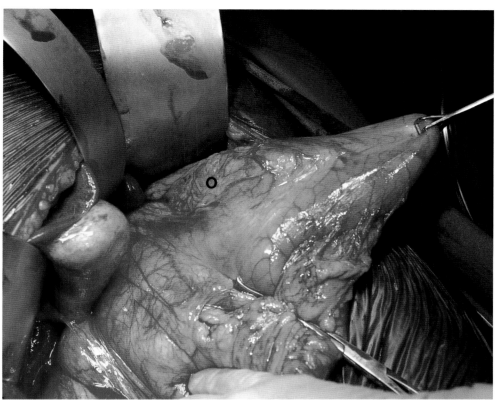

**45** The stomach has been lifted up by the surgeon, who is holding the greater curve palpating the nasogastric tube which has been passed by the anaesthetist.

**46** Shows the lesser omentum (O) stretching from the lesser curve of the stomach to the fissure for the ligamentum venosum of the liver. In the free right hand edge of the lesser omentum lie the common bile duct, hepatic artery and portal vein.

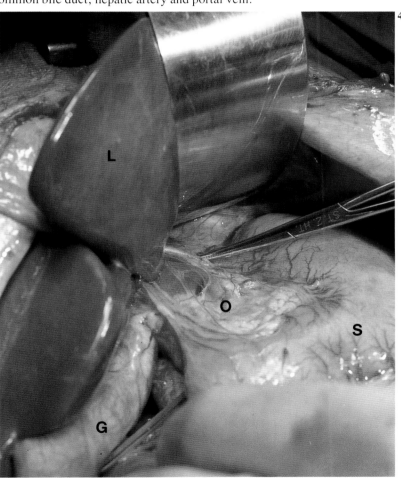

Passing further up, the omentum is attached to the greater curve of the stomach which is yellowish-grey in colour, with a thick wall that can be felt between the fingers. If present, a nasogastric tube can be palpated and its position checked (**45**). The hand is passed to the lesser curve of the stomach and up and to the right on to the *lesser omentum* (**46, 47**). This leads above to the junction of the medial and lateral segments of the left lobe of the liver, which feels solid with a smooth surface and is brownish red in colour.

**47** View of the lesser omentum (O) with the liver (L) lifted up. An anomalous left hepatic artery indicated by the forceps is arising from the left gastric artery. Gall bladder (G), stomach (S).

The left lateral segment of the liver is that part of the organ lying to the left of the *ligamentum teres* and *falciform ligaments* and the fissure containing the embryological remnant of the ligamentum venosum, into which the lesser omentum is attached (**48**). The left lateral segment is suspended from the diaphragm by the left triangular ligament, lying in front of the intra-abdominal oesophagus (**49**).

The hand is then passed across the oesophagus to the fundus of the stomach and to the left of the upper part of the greater curve where the short gastric vessels pass to the stomach from the *hilum of the spleen* in the gastro-splenic ligament (**50**). The spleen is rounded in shape, firm, friable and brick red in colour (**51**). It nestles under the left cupola of the diaphragm which lies between it and the ninth, tenth and eleventh left ribs. Its mobility is restricted by peritoneal and vascular attachments and it can be easily torn during surgery by inappropriate retraction. Below and behind the spleen can be felt the left kidney, recognised by its firm consistency and characteristic bean-shaped outline. Lying behind the posterior parietal peritoneum it cannot be seen or fully examined without deliberate mobilisation.

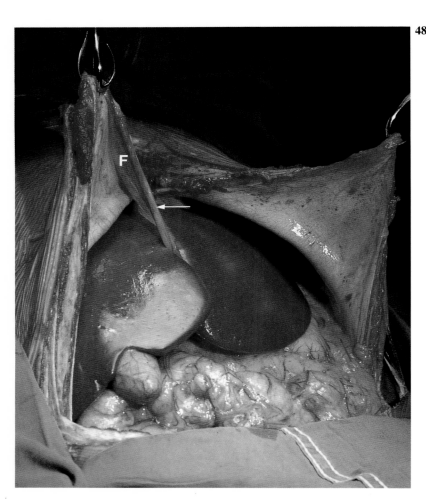

**48**  Shows the falciform ligament of the liver (F), separating the left lateral segment of the left lobe from the left medial segment. The ligamentum teres (arrow) runs in the free edge of the falciform ligament and is the remnant of the foetal umbilical vein.

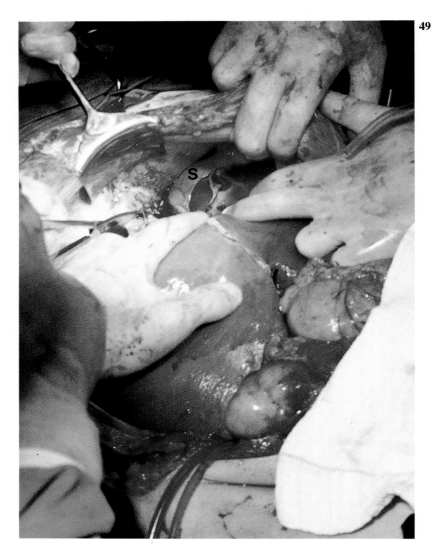

**49**  The falciform ligament of the liver has been cut and the diaphragm can be seen to the left where the stomach (S) is nestling under the costal margin. This picture is of a liver transplant, the liver has been perfused to cool it and remove its contained blood. It is therefore pale in colour, although still alive.

The hand is then brought anterior from the surface of the kidney to the inferior extremity of the spleen and onto the *splenic flexure* of the colon which is attached to the diaphragm by the *phrenicocolic ligament*. The large bowel can be traced in continuity with the transverse colon already seen and the *descending colon* passing down the left side of the abdomen. The descending colon can be palpated *in situ* since it bulges forwards from behind the posterior parietal peritoneum, but it cannot be lifted up like the transverse colon because it has no mesentery. It lies in front of the left kidney and the gas contained in it imparts a resonant note to percussion over the front of the kidney. At the pelvic brim it becomes the *pelvic* or *sigmoid colon*, which is mobile with a mesentery containing branches of the inferior mesenteric vessels (**52**). It is of variable length and diameter but is typically about 30 cm long and resembles the transverse colon. It leads to the *rectum* in the midline which lies in the hollow of the sacrum, passing in the sacral concavity, behind the pelvic peritoneum to join the *anus*.

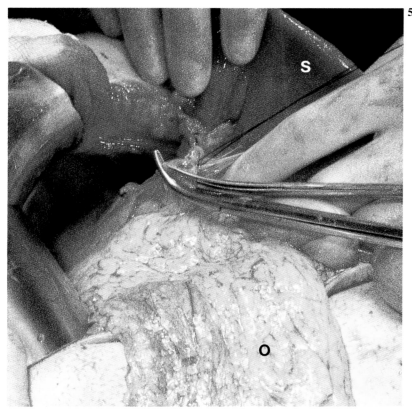

**50** Shows the mobilised spleen (S) and clamps on the short gastric vessels which have been divided between the hilum of the spleen and the greater curve of the stomach. The omentum (O) is hanging downward in the middle of the picture.

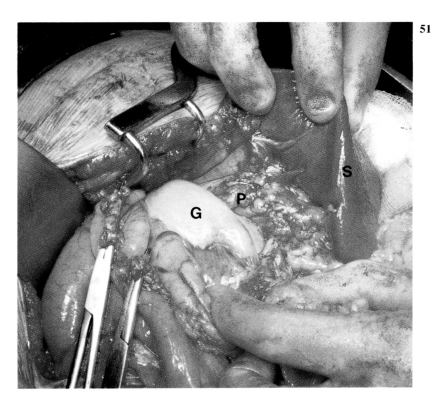

**51** The spleen (S) has now been separated from the greater curve of the stomach (G) and the tail of the pancreas (P) can be seen between stomach and spleen.

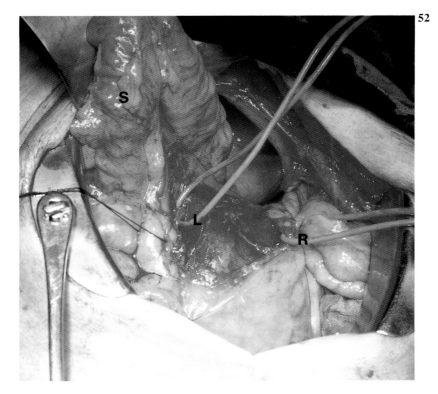

**52** Shows the mobilised pelvic sigmoid colon (S), with a considerable amount of pericolic fat and appendices epiploicae. The view is taken from above, looking towards the pelvis. The red rubber slings control the left and right ureters (L, R). The black silk tie is around the inferior mesenteric artery supplying the pelvic colon.

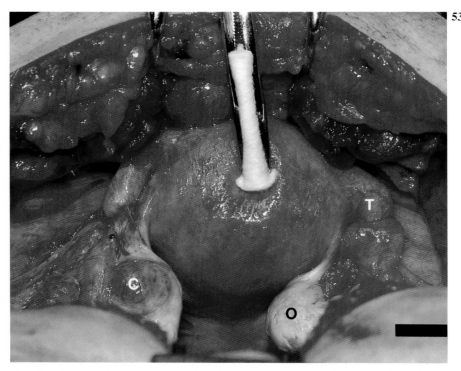

In the female, anterior to the rectum is the vagina below, and the uterus above with a peritoneal cul-de-sac between the two, called the *recto-uterine* pouch of Douglas*, from which peritoneum passes on to the *cervix* and *uterus* and posterior fornix of the vagina. The uterus can now be felt and seen. In the male the recto-vesical pouch is shallow since the partition between the rectum and the prostate is obliterated *in utero* by fusion of the anterior and posterior layers to form the *recto-vesical fascia* of Denonvilliers†. The *fallopian tubes*‡ lie at the upper extremity of the *broad ligaments* and the ovaries are tucked behind the fimbriated ends of the tubes (**53**). Anterior to the vagina and cervix lies the bladder, an extraperitoneal smooth muscular viscus which relaxes to accommodate within limits, whatever urine reaches it from the ureters (**54, 55**). As it fills it pushes the anterior parietal peritoneum up to lie between it and the anterior abdominal wall, where it is more vulnerable to injury than when it is empty and lying protected in the pelvis.

**53** The fundus of the uterus looking down into the pelvis. The fallopian tubes (T) pass backwards towards the pale ovaries (O). There is a follicular cyst (C) on the surface of the left ovary.

**54** Intravenous urogram showing normal appearance of both kidneys (K) and ureters (U) and collection of opacified urine in the bladder (B).

**55** After micturition the bladder has emptied completely. There is no residual urine.

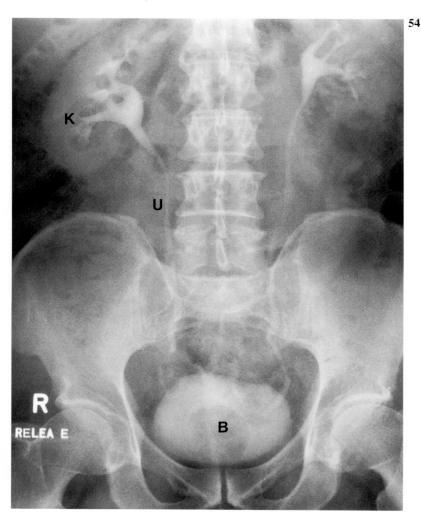

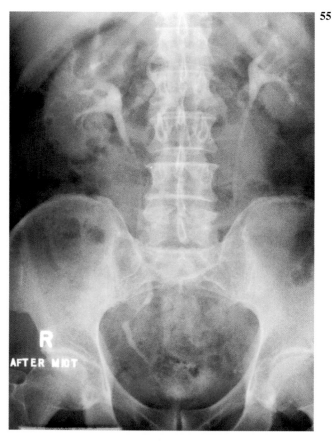

* Douglas, James (1675-1742) Anatomist, male midwife and physician to Queen Caroline, wife of George II.
† Denonvilliers, Charles Pierre (1808-1872) Professor of Anatomy and Surgery – Paris.
‡ Fallopio, Gabriel (1523-1563) Professor of Surgery, Anatomy and Botany – Padua.

The hand is now passed along the pelvic brim. The *aortic bifurcation*, the *common iliac arteries* and their bifurcations into *internal* and *external iliac arteries* can be felt pulsating (**56**). At the points of bifurcation of the common iliac arteries, the ureters cross in front, passing in the retroperitoneal space, lateral to the vertebral bodies *en route* to the base of the bladder deep in the pelvis (**57**). A writhing peristalsis (vermiculation) of the ureters can often be seen but if quiescent when inspected, gentle pressure with forceps will stimulate this vermiform movement, which is a unique characteristic of the ureters and therefore identifies them with certainty. The ureters pass medially and downwards towards the base of the bladder entering the *trigone* of the bladder in the pelvis. The *gonadal vessels* pass anterior to the ureters and the *vasa deferentia* in the male, loop over the ureters on their way from the internal inguinal rings to the *seminal vesicles*.

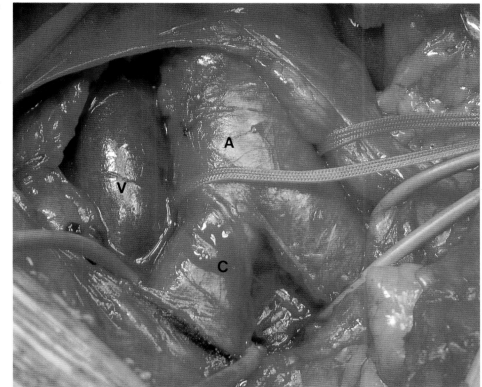

**56**   Shows the bifurcation of the aorta (A) with a tape around it. The right edge of the aorta overlies the left edge of the vena cava (V), which is a dark blue colour and is formed just behind the origin of the right common iliac artery (C).

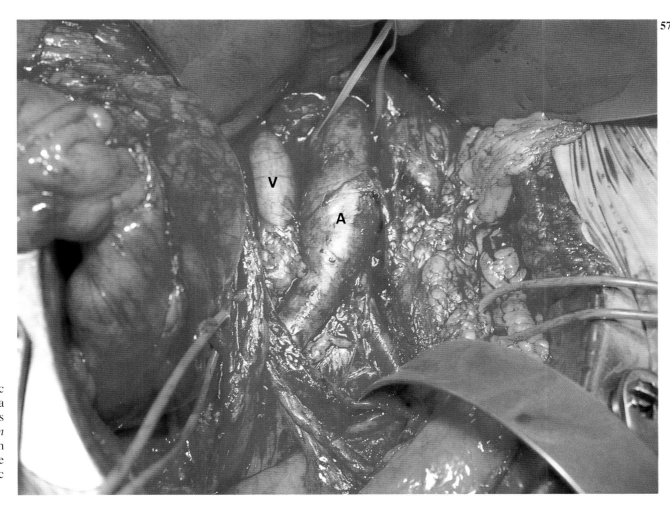

**57**   Another view of the aortic bifurcation (A) and the vena cava (V), showing red rubber slings around the right and left ureters *en route* towards the pelvic brim which they cross in front of the division of the common iliac arteries.

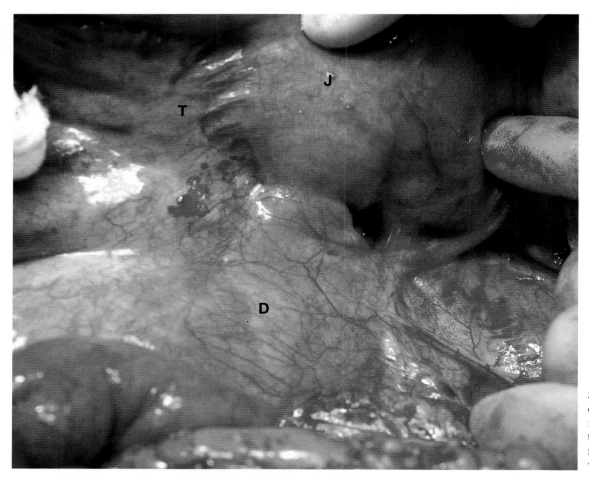

**58** Shows the duodeno-jejunal flexure, the duodenum (D) is retroperitoneal, the jejunum (J) is mobile on its mesentery. The peritoneal fold on the convexity of the flexure contains a smooth muscle band called the ligament of Treitz (T) which passes up to the left crus of the diaphragm.

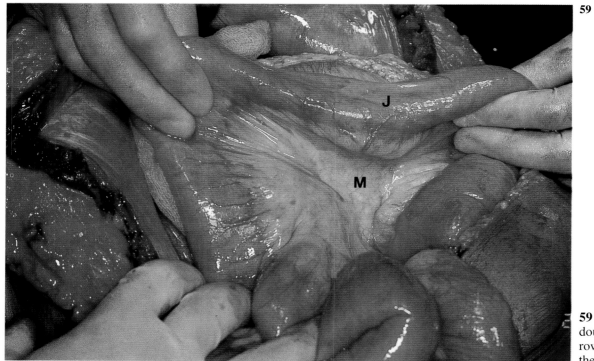

**59** Shows a loop of jejunum (J). The wall has a double feel to it. The mesentery (M) contains one row of vascular arcades. Fat does not encroach on the bowel wall.

The aortic bifurcation can be felt in front of the fourth lumbar vertebra and lies on the origin of the inferior vena cava which is soft, collapsible and blue in colour. All the major vessels lie behind the posterior parietal peritoneum. The hand is now passed into the right iliac fossa. The whole of the small bowel lying in loose coils passes up and to the left to its origin at the *duodeno-jejunal flexure* (**58**), which is the point where the small bowel emerges from the retroperitoneal space into the abdominal cavity. The band of peritoneum containing the *ligament of Treitz**, holds the duodeno-jejunal flexure in place. The loops of small bowel can be lifted up showing the vascular arcades from the superior mesenteric vessels (**59, 60**). The root of the small bowel mesentery is followed from the upper left, across the midline to the lower right where the ileum joins the baggy *caecum*. The caecum resembles a pouch where the taeniae coli converge to the base of the *vermiform appendix*, which arises as a finger-like appendage of the caecum, of variable length, usually about 10 cm long and 8 mm in diameter with its own mesentery (**61**). The appendix may lie pointing in any direction in the peritoneal cavity or behind the caecum.

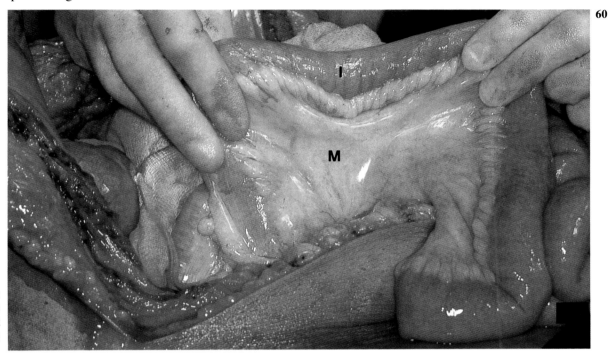

**60** Shows a loop of ileum (I), which feels single and thinner than the jejunum. There are two or three rows of vascular arcades. Fat encroaches from the mesentery (M) onto the wall of the bowel.

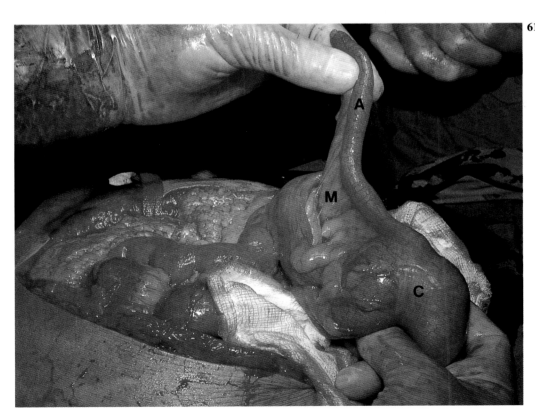

**61** Shows the appendix (A) and mobilised caecum (C). The appendicular artery runs in the small mesentery of the appendix (M). It is a branch of the ileocolic which is the terminal branch of the superior mesenteric artery.

* Treitz, Wenzel (1819-1872) Austrian physician and pathologist.

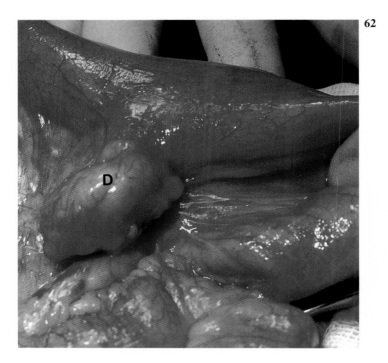

**62**

A vestigial remnant of the embryological vitello-intestinal duct called a Meckel's* diverticulum occurs in 2% of the population approximately 2ft (50cm) from the ileo-caecal junction. It is usually about 2 inches (5cm) in length. It may become inflamed and mimic appendicitis, or develop ulceration due to a lining of ectopic gastric epithelium (**62-65**).

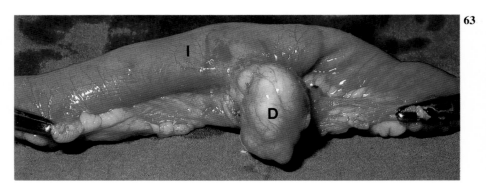

**63**

**62**   Shows a Meckel's diverticulum (D) approximately 50cm from the ileo-caecal junction.

**63**   The loop of ileum (I) containing the Meckel's diverticulum (D) has been removed.

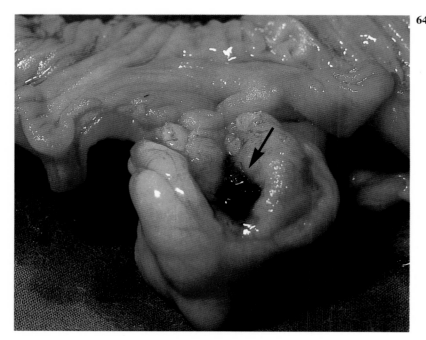

**64**

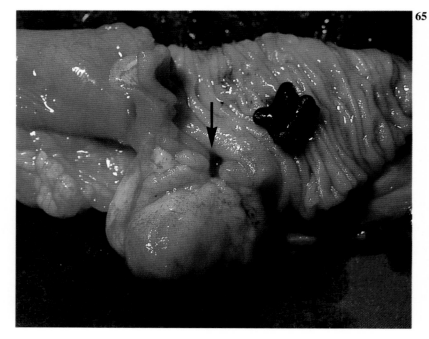

**65**

**64**   The diverticulum has been opened, showing a blood clot lying in an ulcer (arrow). The ulcer lies at the junction of ectopic acid-secreting cell lining and normal columnar cell epithelium of the ileum.

**65**   The clot has been removed from the ulcer cavity (arrow), which can be seen easily.

* Meckel, Johann Friedrich II (1781-1833) Professor of Anatomy – Berlin.

The caecum, partially free in the peritoneal cavity, joins the *ascending colon*, which lies behind the peritoneum. This passes upwards and towards the right lobe of the liver and is a mirror image of the descending colon on the left. It overlies the right kidney and continues as the intra-peritoneal hepatic flexure, leading to the transverse colon. As with the descending colon, the ascending colon also contains gas and therefore percussion of the abdominal wall in front of the right kidney will also have a resonant note. The right lobe and medial segment of the left lobe of the liver can now be seen (**66**). The hand is passed over the convex diaphragmatic surface of the liver to the right of the falciform ligament as far as the anterior layer of the *coronary* and *right triangular ligaments*. The lower edge of the right lobe of the liver is gently lifted up to reveal the under surface which shelves up and posteriorly. The gall bladder is a pear-shaped, baggy viscus with a slightly greenish tinge. It is partially embedded in its fossa in the under surface of the right lobe of the liver.

A plane drawn from the bed of the gall bladder fossa to the vena cava is the true boundary of vascular, biliary and segmental anatomy between the right and left lobes of the liver (**67**). Between the neck of the gall bladder and the pylorus of the stomach is the right, lateral free edge of the lesser omentum containing the *portal vein* posteriorly, the *common bile duct* in front and to the right. The *common hepatic artery* can be felt pulsating anteriorly to the left of the common bile duct.

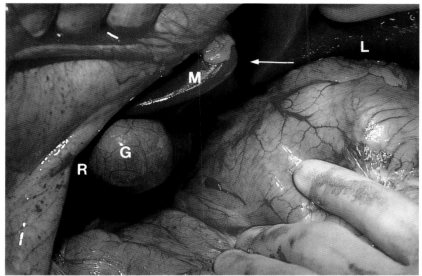

**66** Shows the gall bladder (G) in its fossa. To the left of the gall bladder is the fissure of the ligamentum teres (arrow), separating the left lateral (L) from the left medial segment (M), which extends as far as the gall bladder bed to the right of which is the edge of the right lobe (R). The left index finger of the surgeon is in the middle of Rutherford Morison's pouch.

**67** Diagram of the liver to show the anatomical plane separating the right (R) and left (L) lobes, running from the bed of the gall bladder to the inferior vena cava. Right kidney (K), stomach (G), spleen (S).

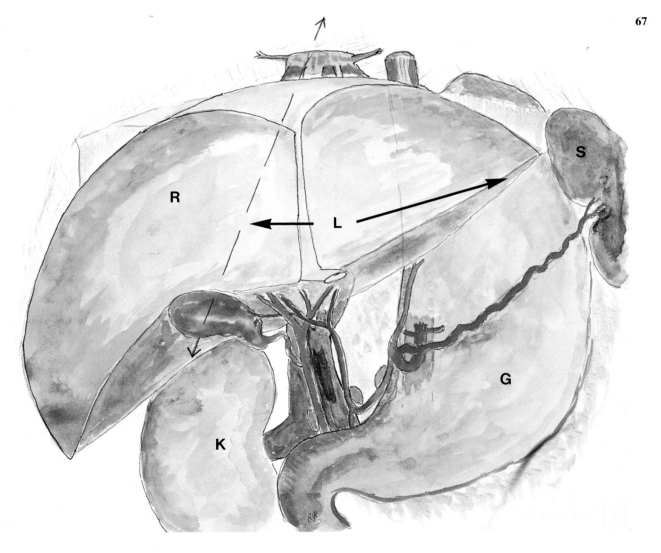

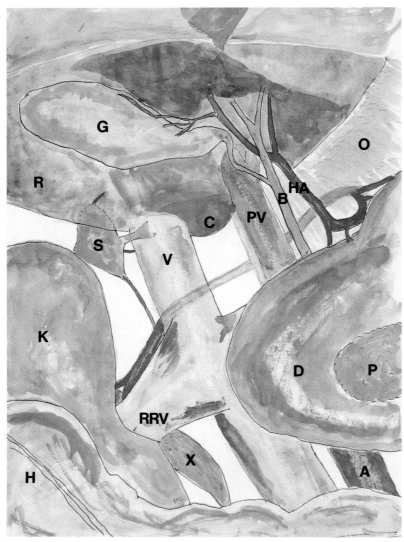

Behind this important peritoneal fold is the opening or *aditus* of the lesser sac. A finger passed through this orifice will have the free edge of the lesser omentum with its vital contents in front, the inferior vena cava behind, the first part of the duodenum below and the caudate process of the caudate lobe of the liver above. Just lateral to the aditus of the lesser sac, the right kidney can be felt, a mirror image of the left. The space below the right lobe of the liver, *Rutherford Morison's\* pouch*, is very important since it is often the site of disease (**68**). It can be regarded as the 'Piccadilly Circus'† for the general surgeon since, if he does not know exactly where he is and take care, he will get into trouble!

Many pathological conditions of surgical interest can involve important organs within a few centimetres of each other, namely the gall bladder, the right lobe of the liver, the first part of the duodenum, the head of the pancreas, the right kidney, the renal pelvis and upper ureter, the inferior vena cava, the right renal artery and vein, the right adrenal gland tucked behind the inferior vena cava and finally the common bile duct, portal vein and hepatic artery.

The above laparotomy tour around the abdominal cavity will enable the surgeon to see or feel most abdominal organs and identify any gross pathological abnormalities by a combination of vision and touch. Assessment of structures behind the posterior parietal peritoneum will not have been completed until the posterior peritoneum is opened to permit more direct access. Assessment of the pancreas requires opening the *lesser sac* and mobilisation of the first and second parts of the duodenum. The peritoneum, lateral to the second part of the duodenum, is incised and blunt finger dissection beyond the vena cava as far as the abdominal aorta permits elevation of the duodenal 'C' around the head of the pancreas (**69, 70**). This is known as Kocher's‡ manoeuvre

**68** Diagram of the subhepatic space of Rutherford Morison showing the proximity of vital structures to each other in this site, the 'Piccadilly Circus' of the abdomen. Right lobe of liver (R), gall bladder (G), caudate process (C), lesser omentum (O), duodenum (D), head of pancreas (P), aorta (A), inferior vena cava (V), right kidney (K), right adrenal (S), hepatic flexure of colon (H), portal vein (PV), common bile duct (B), hepatic artery (HA), right renal vein (RRV), renal pelvis (X).

**69**

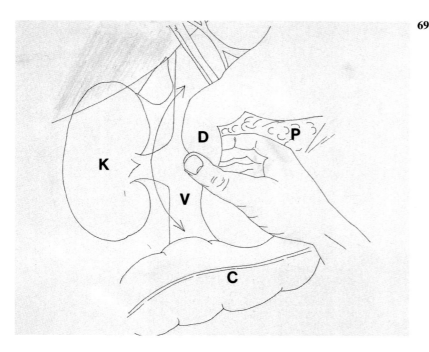

**69** Kocher's manoeuvre. An incision has been made in the peritoneum lateral to the convexity of the C-curve of the duodenum (D) which is lifted up. Right kidney (K), inferior vena cava (V), pancreas (P), transverse colon (C).

\* Morison, James Rutherford (1853-1939) Newcastle surgeon.
† Equivalent to Times Square.
‡ Kocher, Emil Theodor (1841-1917) Professor of Surgery – Berne – the first surgeon to be awarded the Nobel Prize (1909), for his studies of the thyroid gland.

**70** Shows the structures revealed when an extensive Kocher's manoeuvre has been performed in an organ donor operation. The vena cava (V) and aorta (A) are clearly seen. The right ureter lying on the green towel has been cut (arrow). Right kidney (K), gall bladder (G), duodenum (D), ascending colon (C), appendix (X), caecum (Y).

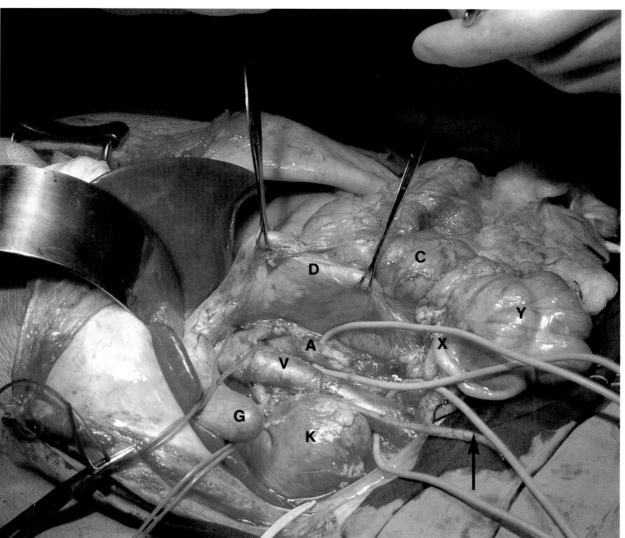

If the greater omentum is divided between the gastro-epiploic vascular arcade and the transverse colon, the stomach can be lifted up and the colon pushed down exposing the front of the body and tail of the pancreas (**71–73**). The surgeon's right hand is passed in the lesser sac up behind the oesophagus to assess the oesophageal hiatus in the diaphragm and palpate the upper abdominal aorta.

Most of the important surgical, anatomical features can be appreciated without causing harm to the patient by careful laparotomy, Kocher's manoeuvre and opening the lesser sac.

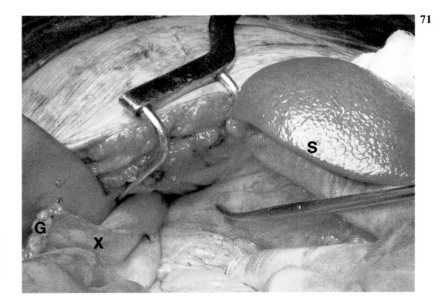

**71** Shows the lesser sac after division of the short gastric vessels (G) and part of the greater omentum from the greater curve of the stomach. The forceps points to the pancreas. The stomach (X) can be seen on the right and the spleen (S) on the left.

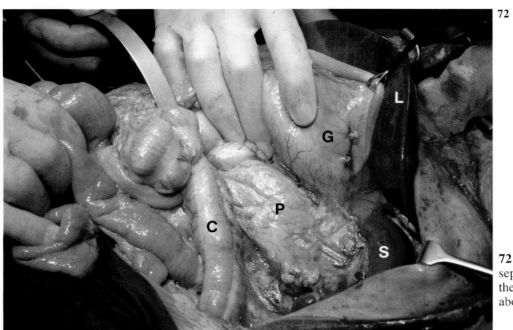

**72** The greater curve of the stomach (G) has been elevated and separated from the transverse colon (C). The pancreas (P) lies in the lesser sac, the spleen can be seen to the left (S) and the liver (L) above the stomach.

**73** Closer view of same field shown in **72**.

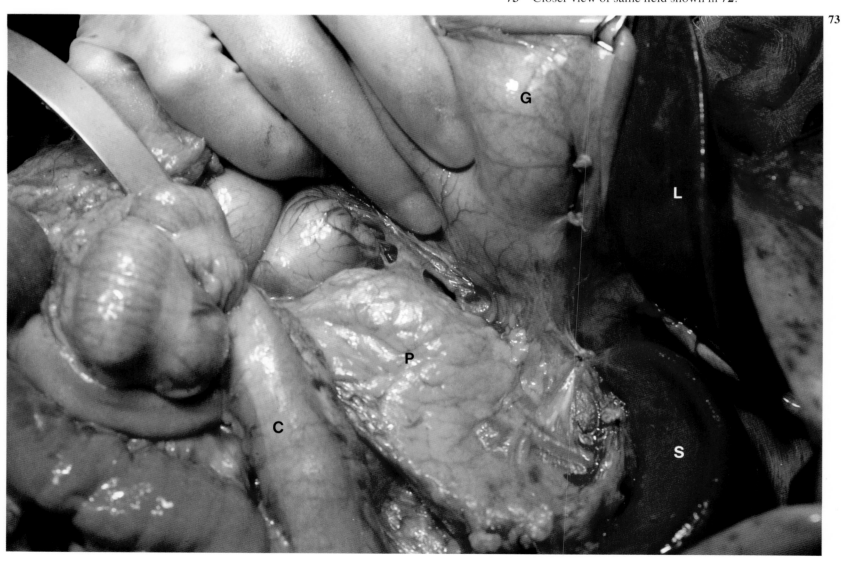

# 2 The Abdominal Wall, Herniae, External Genitalia, Perineum, Diaphragm, Nerves Entering and Leaving the Abdomen

## The Abdominal Wall

Three layers of muscle, the external and internal oblique and the transversus, pass from the rib cage to the pelvis extending posteriorly from the quadratus lumborum loin muscles forwards towards the midline (74). Here they fuse to form a sheath, which encloses the strong strap-shaped rectus abdominis muscles which also pass from the chest to the pelvis. All these muscles are innervated segmentally by the intercostal nerves T7 to T12 and L1 which lie between the internal oblique and transversus. The detailed attachments of the muscles are seldom of importance in surgical practice, but the external oblique is the key muscle in the anatomy of herniae.

The abdomen is usually approached surgically through the anterior abdominal wall with a median or a paramedian incision (75). The scalpel cuts through skin, superficial fascia and its fibrous deep component, *Scarpa's fascia**, which passes down into the scrotum as Colles fascia†. There is no deep fascia over the abdominal wall. In the midline the fibrous aponeuroses of the muscles are fused to form a tough band, the linea alba, which when cut, leads straight into the peritoneal cavity. In a paramedian incision the anterior rectus sheath is incised and the rectus muscle is freed from the sheath medially by cutting the anterior fibrous intersections between the muscle and the sheath.

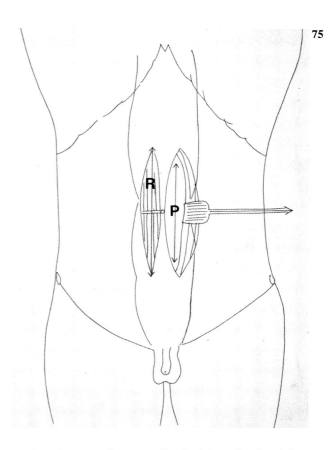

**75** Diagram of paramedian incision. On the right a longitudinal incision has been made through the skin, subcutaneous tissue and anterior rectus sheath to reveal the rectus abdominus muscle (R). On the left the tendinous intersection has been divided so that the rectus muscle can be retracted laterally as shown. The posterior rectus sheath (P) is then incised longitudinally.

**74** CT scan of the abdomen showing the three layers of the abdominal muscle (arrow), namely external oblique, internal oblique and transversus, laterally and the two recti muscles (R) anteriorly. Psoas muscle (P) can be seen on each side of the vertebral body. Quadratus lumborum (q), and erector spinae (e,s) are also shown.

* Scarpa, Antonio (1747-1832) Professor of Anatomy – Padua.
† Colles, Abraham (1773-1843) Surgeon – Dublin.

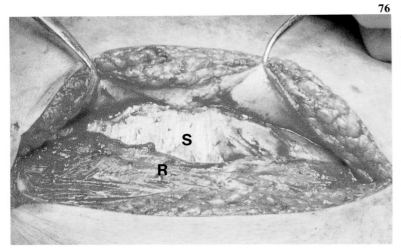

**76** Shows a paramedian incision. The rectus muscle (R) has been retracted laterally and the posterior rectus sheath (S) will be incised longitudinally.

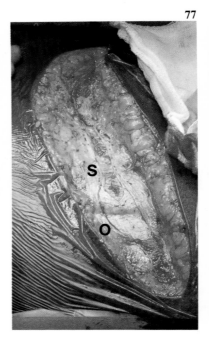

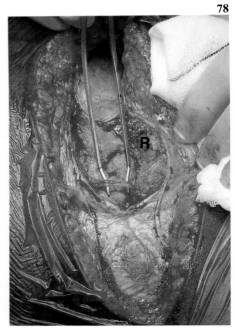

The muscle is then pulled laterally and the posterior rectus sheath cut to open the peritoneal cavity (**76**). Since many other incisions may be indicated under special circumstances (**77-80**), a brief description of the muscles of the abdominal wall is necessary and will include the anatomy of inguinal and femoral herniae.

**77** Right subcostal (Kocher's) incision: the skin and subcutaneous tissue have been divided and the external oblique (O) and anterior rectus sheath (S) have been incised.

**78** Continuation of the subcostal incision. The rectus muscle (R) has been divided as has the external oblique and part of the internal oblique. The forceps demonstrate the ninth intercostal nerve, which lies between the internal oblique and transversus muscles and passes into the rectus sheath to supply the rectus muscle.

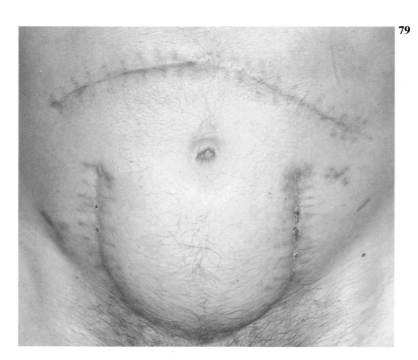

**79** Shows a bilateral subcostal incision and iliac fossa incisions, the former to approach the kidneys, the latter the iliac vessels.

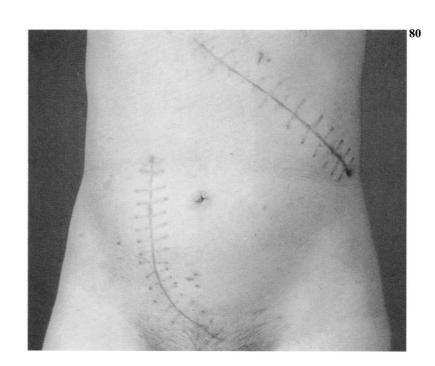

**80** Shows a left subcostal incision and a right iliac fossa incision, the former to approach the spleen and the latter the iliac vessels.

*The external oblique* arises from the outer surface of the lower eight ribs interdigitating with the origin of the *serratus anterior* above and the *latissimus dorsi* below. The lower fibres pass down to the iliac crest whilst the remaining fibres pass downwards medially and become incorporated into a tough fibrous sheet, the aponeurosis. This forms the anterior layer of the rectus sheath medially whilst below it is fixed to the *anterior superior iliac spine* and *pubic tubercle*. Between these two points it is stretched as an upward looking, gutter shaped band, the *inguinal ligament of Poupart**, bound distally to the deep *fascia lata* of the thigh (**81-83**).

The inguinal ligament is a key structure in the anatomy of herniae. The fibres of the ligament attached to the pubic tubercle continue posteriorly as the sickle shaped, *lacunar ligament of Gimbernat*†, also poorly named the *pectineal part of the inguinal ligament*. The fibres continue laterally over the origin of the pectineus muscle to join the pectineal line of the superior pubic ramus as the *pectineal ligament of Astley Cooper*‡.

*The internal oblique* arises from the lumbar fascia, iliac crest and lateral half of the curved deep edge of the inguinal ligament. Its fibres pass up and medially at right angles to those of the external oblique.

**81**

**82**

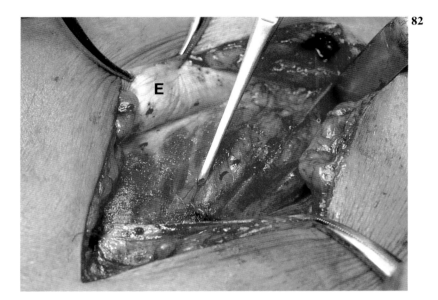

**82** Operation for right inguinal hernia. The external oblique aponeurosis (E) had been divided and turned back to show the fibres of the internal oblique to which the forceps are pointing.

**81** Diagram of the external abdominal muscles. On the right the external oblique (E) is shown, passing from above and laterally to below and medially where the aponeurosis forms the inguinal ligament below and the anterior portion of the anterior rectus sheath (S) medially. On the left is shown the internal oblique muscle (I). Its fibres pass from below upwards and medially. This muscle forms part of the conjoint tendon and the deep layer of the anterior rectus sheath and the superficial layer of posterior rectus sheath.

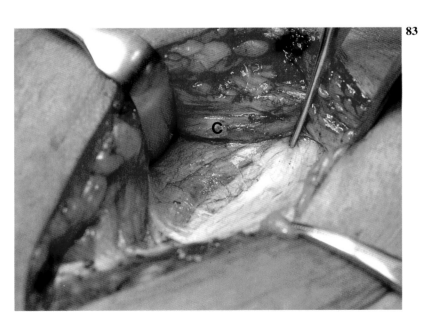

**83** Further dissection of the inguinal canal. The spermatic cord (C) has been retracted upwards and to the left and the instrument points to where the white fibres of the inguinal ligament are attached medially to the pubic tubercle.

* Poupart, François (1601-1709) Surgeon and Naturalist – Paris.
† Gimbernat, y Arbos (1734-1816) Surgeon and Professor of Anatomy – Barcelona.
‡ Cooper, Sir Astley Paston (1768-1841) Surgeon of Guy's and St Thomas's Hospitals – London.

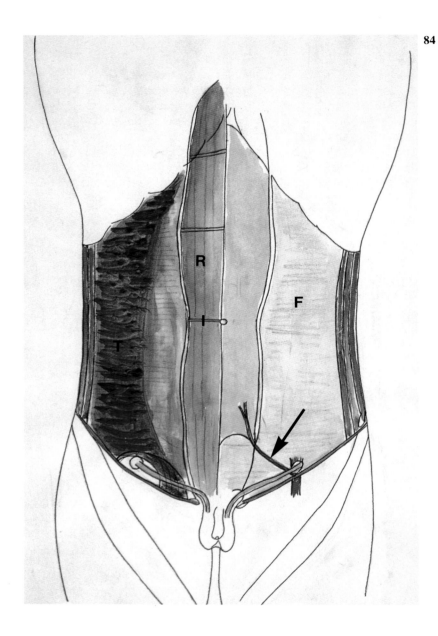

**84** The posterior fibres are inserted into the 10th, 11th and 12th ribs and costal cartilages. Above and medially it also forms an aponeurosis. This splits into anterior and posterior layers. The former fused with the external oblique completes the anterior layer of the rectus sheath. The latter passes behind the rectus muscle in its upper two thirds, except over the costal cartilage where there is no posterior rectus sheath. There is also no posterior rectus sheath in the lower third, where the lower medial portion of the internal oblique swings downwards, helping to form an arch over the lateral part of the inguinal canal, which passes behind the medial part of the inguinal canal to join the pubic crest and pectineal line of the superior pubic ramus. This is the internal oblique's contribution to the *conjoint tendon*, misnamed since it is composed mainly of muscle fibres not collagen.

*The transversus* arises from the seventh to twelfth costal cartilages interdigitating with fibres of the diaphragm and from the lumbar fascia that encloses the quadratus lumborum, the anterior two thirds of the inner lip of the iliac crest and the lateral third of the inguinal ligament. It passes transversely across the lateral part of the abdomen (**84**). Above and medially muscle fibres lie behind the internal oblique's contribution to the posterior rectus sheath until close to the midline an aponeurosis is formed which fuses with the linea alba. In the middle the aponeurosis is more extensive, strengthening the posterior rectus sheath. Below the muscle fibres form in an arch to fuse with fibres of the internal oblique to form the conjoint tendon.

*The rectus muscles* On each side of the linea alba are the strong strap like muscles arising from the *xiphoid process* and the fifth, sixth and seventh costal cartilages. They pass vertically down to the pubic tubercles and crests, each joined by a small wedge shaped muscle, the pyramidalis, which passes from the pubic crest to the linea alba. Each rectus has a tough protective sheath enclosing all but the lowermost portion posteriorly and that part in front of the costal cartilages. The lower limit of the posterior rectus sheath is curved, concave inferiorly (the *arcuate* line).

*The transversalis fascia* is a layer of fibrous connective tissue, less well defined than the muscular aponeuroses, which lies between the transversus muscle and the parietal peritoneum, and continues into the pelvis as the *pelvic fascia*. In the inguinal region it lies behind the inguinal canal and forms part of its posterior wall, being fused with the deep part of the inguinal ligament and extending over the femoral vessels as the *femoral sheath*. An orifice in it at the mid-inguinal point, the internal inguinal ring, allows egress of the *spermatic cord* in the male and the *round ligament* in the female. It is continuous with the *fascia iliaca* overlying the pelvic muscles.

**84** Diagram showing the deeper layers of the anterior abdominal wall. On the right the transversus muscle (T) can be seen. It contributes also to the conjoint tendon and the posterior layer of the rectus sheath. Also shown is the right rectus muscle (R) and the tendinous intersections (I) are indicated. On the left the transversalis fascia (F) is indicated. The inferior epigastric artery (arrow) arising from the external iliac artery can be seen entering the rectus sheath, which is deficient posteriorly in its lower third and uppermost portion over the costal margin.

# Herniae

A hernia is a protrusion of tissue into a place where it should not be. There are many varieties but the majority involve protrusions of the parietal peritoneum.

**A** In relation to the inguinal ligament. The anatomy of these will be considered.

**B** Through or beside the umbilicus, the former in infants, the latter in adults (**85-87**).

**C** At a site of weakness following surgical incisions where muscles may have been denervated or healing impaired by infection or poor surgical technique (**88**).

**D** Through the *oesophageal hiatus* in the diaphragm where the stomach slides up into the chest or rolls up alongside the oesophagus (**89-94**).

**E** Internal herniae. For example into the lesser sac or through a defect in the mesentery.

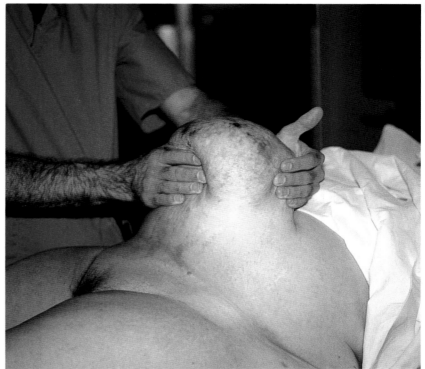

**85** Shows a huge para-umbilical hernia.

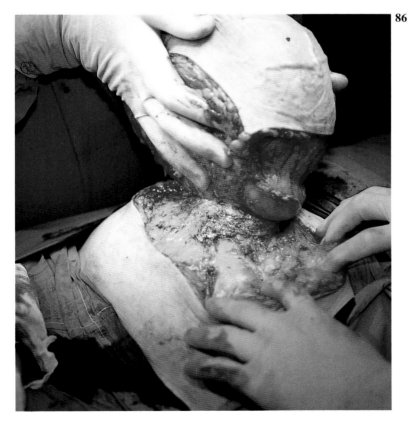

**86** Dissection of the para-umbilical hernia with removal of the overlying skin.

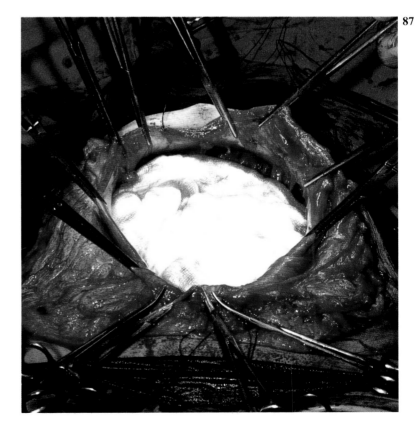

**87** Defect of para-umbilical hernia which will require careful closure with strong unabsorbable material, for example dacron. (White swab in wound.)

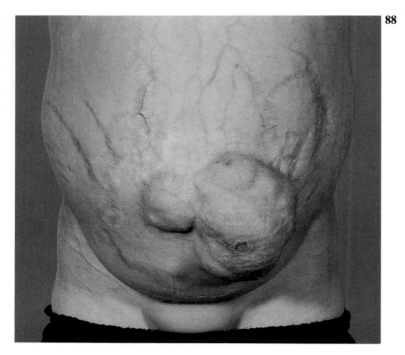

**88**  Incisional hernia in a jaundiced patient treated with steroids which have resulted in the longitudinal striae and also impair wound-healing.

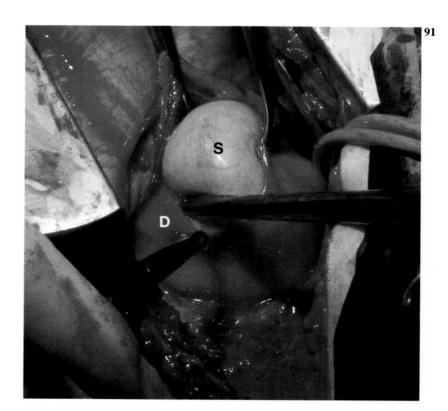

**89**  Diagram of a sliding hiatus hernia. The stomach (S) has entered the chest and brought with it a sac of peritoneum (arrow).

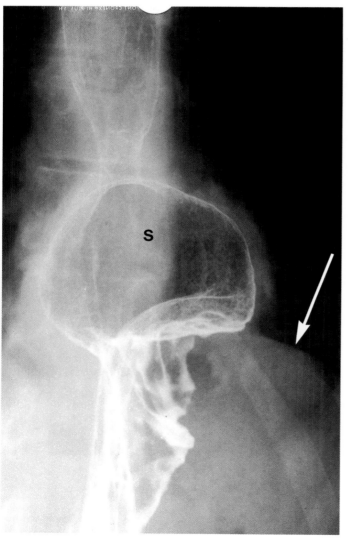

**91**  Operation on a sliding hiatus hernia through the chest. The diaphragm (D) has been incised and the hernial sac opened revealing the light-coloured stomach (S) which will be returned to the abdomen.

**90**  Barium study of a sliding hiatus hernia – the fundus and body of the stomach (S) are above the diaphragm (arrow).

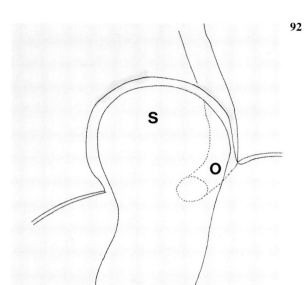

**92** Diagram of a rolling hiatus hernia. The fundus and greater curve of the stomach (S) have rolled into the chest in front of the oesophagus (O).

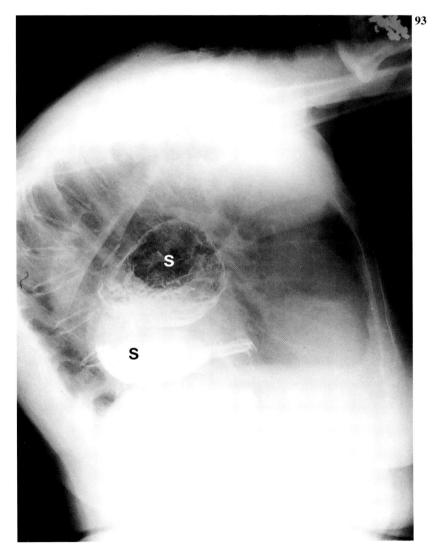

**93** Lateral chest X-ray in a patient who has swallowed barium, showing the whole stomach (S) within the chest. This is a rolling hiatus hernia.

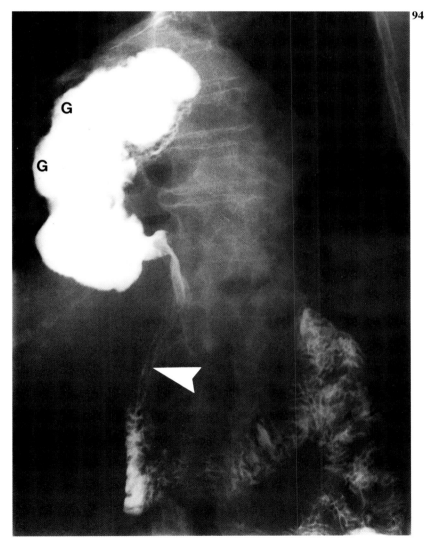

**94** Barium study of rolling hiatus hernia. The greater curve (G) has rotated up into the chest; the duodenum is seen below (arrow).

*Inguinal and femoral herniae*. During intra-uterine development, in the course of its descent from the posterior abdominal wall, the testis passes through the inguinal canal and descends into the scrotum trailing its blood supply from the aorta and its duct, the *vas deferens*, from the *prostatic urethra*. It also brings nerves and lymphatics and with it the *processus vaginalis*, an outpouching of the peritoneal cavity which picks up three coverings *en route*:

**A** the *internal spermatic fascia* from the fascia transversalis;
**B** the cremasteric muscle from the internal oblique, supplied by the genital branch of the genito-femoral nerve, L1 and 2;
**C** the *external spermatic fascia* from the external oblique.

The processus vaginalis pouch becomes cut off from the main peritoneal cavity to form a separate enclosure for the testis, the *tunica vaginalis*. A hydrocoele is an excessive collection of fluid in the tunica vaginalis.

The foetal connection of the scrotum can persist as a *patent processus vaginalis* or a new peritoneal sac can be pushed anterior to the spermatic cord or round ligament (**95, 96**). These are both herniae with oblique courses, called indirect inguinal herniae, which differentiates them from direct inguinal herniae which pass directly forwards through the posterior wall of the inguinal canal. Direct herniae occur most often in elderly men with weak abdominal muscles.

**95** Diagram of an obstructed inguinal hernia in which a loop of ileum has entered an oblique hernial sac and has been obstructed at the neck (arrow) of the hernia so that the small bowel proximal (P) to the obstruction is grossly dilated and the small bowel distal (D) is collapsed and shrunken.

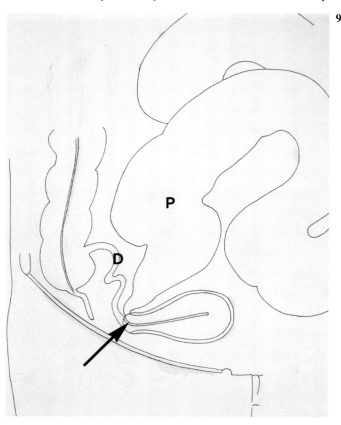

**95**

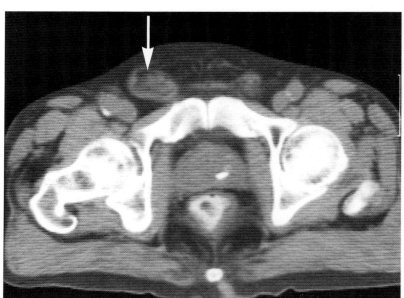

**96**

**96** A CT scan showing an inguinal hernia on the right side, indicated by the arrow. Excess fat (omentum) has entered the canal.

**97**

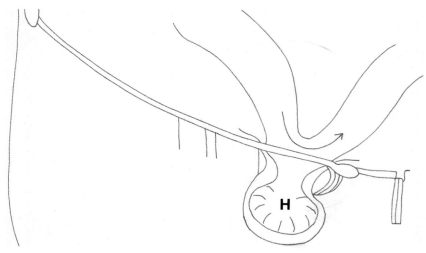

**98**

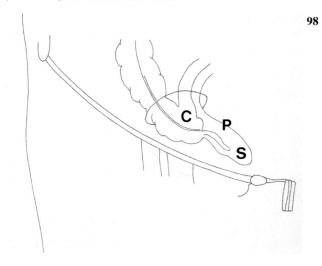

**97** Diagram of a Richter's* femoral hernia showing that only part of the bowel wall thickness has entered the hernia (H), where strangulation and rupture can occur without obstruction taking place. The patient may present with dangerous generalised peritonitis and little in the way of preceding symptoms.

**98** Diagram of a sliding inguinal hernia in which the sac (S) consists partly of parietal peritoneum (P) and partly of visceral peritoneum covering the caecum (C). In repairing such a hernia it is important that the wall of the bowel does not get damaged.

*Richter, August Gottlieb (1742-1812) Surgeon – Göttingen, West Germany.

*Femoral herniae* are less common than inguinal herniae and occur more often in women than men. They pass along the medial side of the femoral vein through the femoral canal (**97**). The peritoneal sac may have extra-peritoneal fat outside it. It may be empty or contain omentum or small bowel.

Colon or bladder with only partial covering of peritoneum may form part of the hernial sac, due to their parietal extra-peritoneal situations. Such a *sliding hernia* may be difficult to repair and the viscus in the wall of the sac if not recognised, may be damaged (**98**).

All the herniae mentioned above are usually repaired by utilising the inguinal ligament as a fixed structure which will hold sutures. A rare but unpleasant hernia, passes in front of the femoral vessels, behind a weakened or damaged inguinal ligament, usually the result of previous surgery. Since the blood vessels must not be damaged

there is little in the way of strong tissue available around the margins of the sac of this *pre-vascular hernia* to permit a sound repair.

It is important to appreciate the three-dimensional obliquity of the inguinal canal from the deep to the superficial and from lateral to medial. The anatomy of groin herniae may be illustrated by imagining that you are walking the course of a hernia (**99**). *Inguinal hernia* – you, an oblique inguinal sac, leave the abdomen alongside the spermatic cord through the internal inguinal ring orifice in the transversalis fascia. Deep to you can be felt the pulsation of the external iliac artery. As you walk medially forwards and downwards, treading on the inguinal ligament, the *inferior epigastric artery* will pass up from the external iliac immediately medial to you, en route for the posterior surface of the rectus abdominis muscle. Beyond this vessel, the transversalis fascia forms the posterior wall of the inguinal

**99**

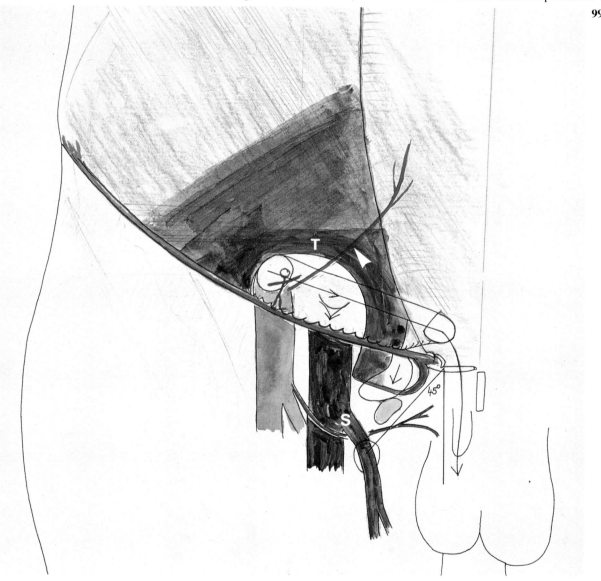

**99** A diagram of the anatomy of inguinal and femoral hernias. The inguinal canal is shown stretching from the deep internal inguinal ring to the superficial external inguinal ring. In traversing the canal, one would first see the conjoint tendon (T), superficial and then arching above the canal, to be inserted posteriorly and deep. The inferior epigastric artery passes around the medial extremity of the internal ring. A direct hernia would appear in the posterior wall medial to the inferior epigastric artery. An oblique indirect hernia arises lateral to the inferior epigastric artery (arrow) and may appear in the groin and

descend into the scrotum. A femoral hernia passes down the femoral canal bounded superficially by the inguinal ligament, medially by the lacunar ligament, posteriorly by Astley Cooper's ligament and laterally by the femoral vein. A lymph node in this situation, named after Cloquet, may if it is inflamed, mimic a femoral hernia. A femoral hernia may present through the saphenous cribriform opening, where the saphenous vein (S) passes deep to join the femoral vein. Inferior to the saphenous vein is the superficial external pudendal artery.

canal and it is through this area that a direct inguinal hernia will reach the inguinal canal. In front of you are the muscle fibres of the conjoint tendon arising from the internal oblique and transversus.

This muscle bundle will arch over your head obliquely to be inserted into the pubic crest and pectineal line of the superior pubic ramus behind you in the lower part of the canal where the external oblique aponeurosis lies directly in front of you. You will emerge from the inguinal canal via the external inguinal ring, a defect in the external oblique, just above, medial and superficial to the pubic tubercle. You are now in the subcutaneous tissue. If you continue to follow the spermatic cord you will reach the scrotum and come to lie in front of the testicle. If you turn upwards, medially in the subcutaneous tissue you reach the commonest site for an *ectopic testis*, called the *superficial inguinal pouch* (**100**).

*Femoral hernia*. You, the sac, push your way through the transversalis fascia, medial to and alongside the femoral vein. In front of you is the tight inguinal ligament which you duck beneath. As you trace this to your medial side you encounter the sharp edge of *Gimbernat's lacunar* (pectineal part of the inguinal) ligament. Behind you is the condensation of fascia on the rigid pectineal line of the superior pubic ramus, Astley Cooper's pectineal ligament. You may observe a prominent artery in 28% of people, arising from the inferior epigastric branch of the external iliac artery. This *abnormal obturator artery* en route for the obturator canal is an important rare variant since in 3% of patients it lies medial to the neck of a femoral hernia passing along the lacunar ligament and may be damaged during surgery.

Your only companion in this confined space of the femoral canal is *Cloquet's** lymph node* with its afferent and efferent lymphatic vessels. The walls that surround you cannot stretch, except for the soft blood-containing femoral vein, hence the likelihood of the strangulation of a femoral hernia. As you pass into the upper medial thigh, out of this confined space, you will emerge on a line approximately 3 cm below and lateral at 45° to the pubic tubercle. Here you may escape from beneath the tough, deep fascia lata of the femoral triangle, to pass alongside the incoming *saphenous vein* and lymphatics through the saphenous *cribriform opening* into the subcutaneous tissues overlying the vein.

The following illustrations demonstrate the anatomy and principles of repair of an indirect inguinal hernia (**101-118**).

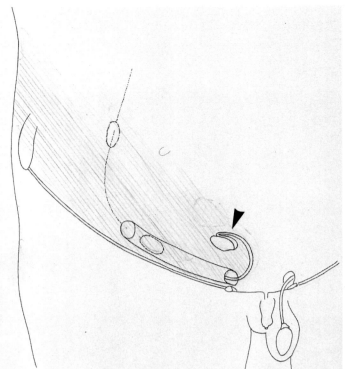

**100** Diagram showing the descent of the testes from the retroperitoneal tissues through the inguinal canal, normally into the scrotum. The most common ectopic situation is shown in the diagram where the testis has come out of the external ring and turned laterally and superficial to lie in the superficial inguinal pouch (arrow).

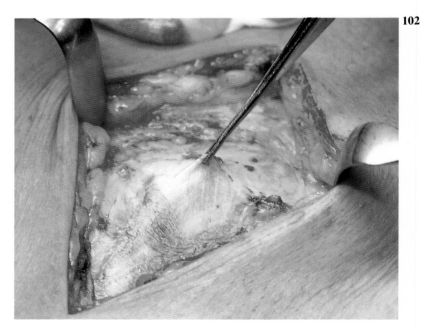

**102** The external oblique aponeurosis is demonstrated and will be cut in the line of the fibres.

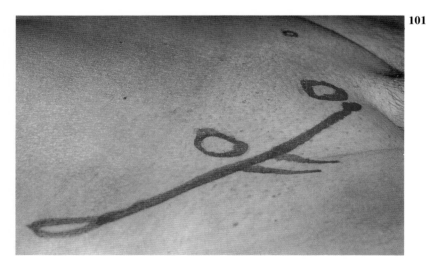

**101** Patient prepared for repair of an oblique inguinal hernia. The inguinal ligament, femoral artery and internal and external inguinal rings are indicated with red ink.

*Cloquet, Baron Jules Germain (1790-1883) Parisian Surgeon to Napoleon III.

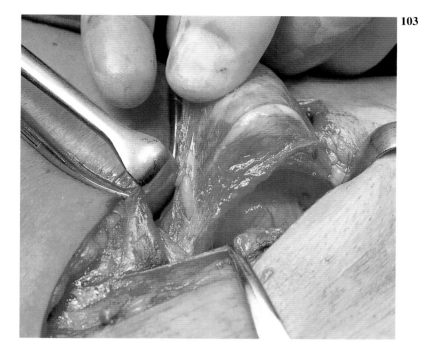

**103** The inguinal canal has been opened and the vas deferens is the white structure under the surgeon's thumb that feels like a piece of string.

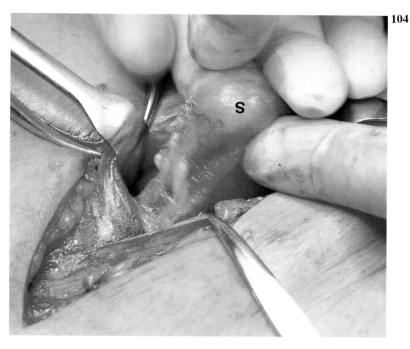

**104** The sac (S) is being separated from the cord.

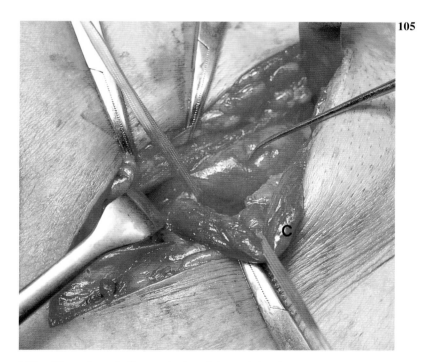

**105** The pointer indicates the hernial sac, it has been separated from the spermatic cord (C) and will be excised.

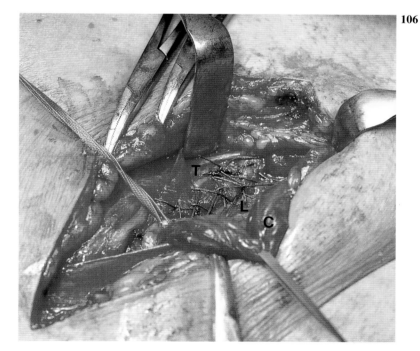

**106** Repair consists of suturing with unabsorbable dacron stitches, the conjoint tendon (T) to the inguinal ligament (L) behind the spermatic cord (C).

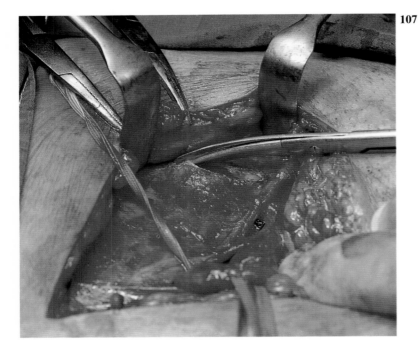

**107** To relieve the tension on the repair an incision is made in the deep layer of the anterior rectus sheath, formed by the internal oblique and transversus muscles (Tanner* slide).

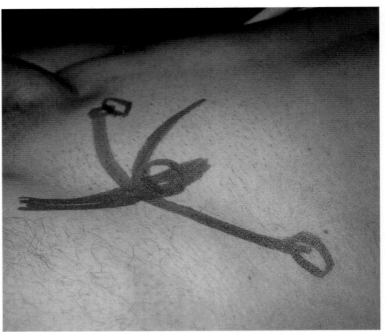

**108** Patient prepared for operation on a left indirect inguinal hernia. The external and internal rings are marked with black ink. The inguinal canal, femoral artery and inferior epigastric artery are marked with red ink.

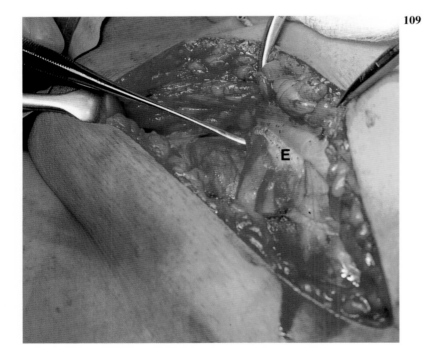

**109** The external oblique aponeurosis (E) has been divided in the line of its fibres.

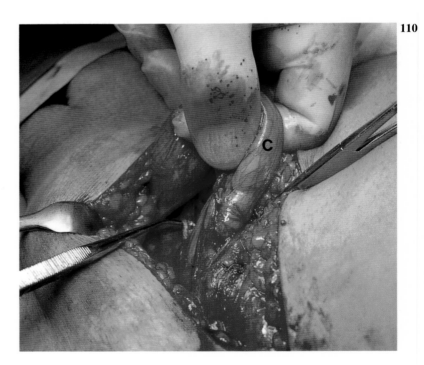

**110** The spermatic cord (C) has been delivered. The pointer is under the ilio-inguinal nerve.

*Tanner, Normal Cecil (1906,1982) London surgeon.

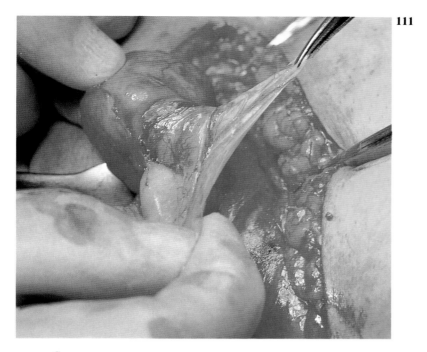

**111** The peritoneal hernial sac has been opened.

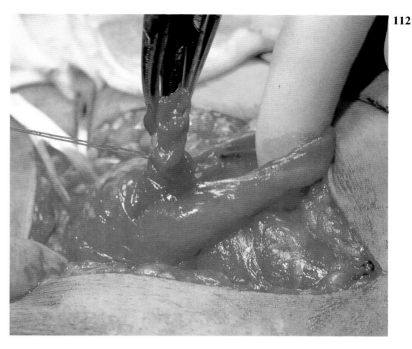

**112** The sac has been twisted and sutured at its neck and the fundus of the sac has been removed.

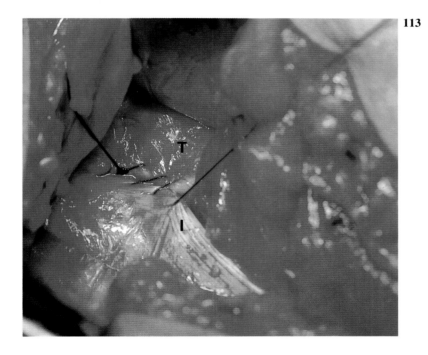

**113** A continuous dacron suture has been inserted between the inguinal ligament (I) and the conjoint tendon (T).

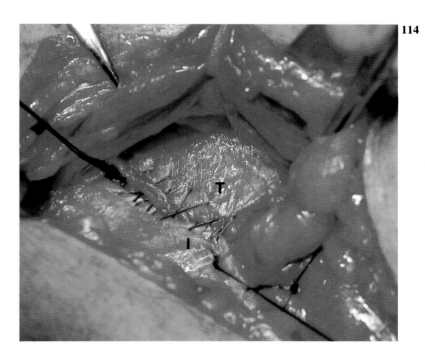

**114** A second layer of sutures completes the repair behind the spermatic cord.

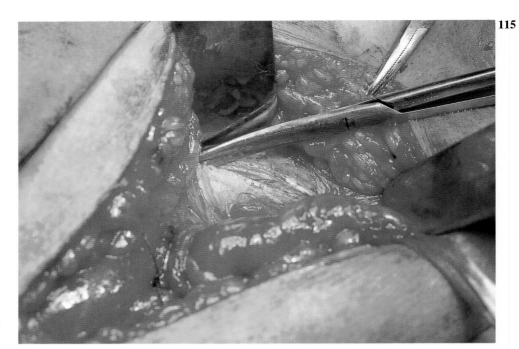

**115** The anterior layer of the anterior rectus sheath is being incised (Tanner slide).

**116** An enormous right oblique inguinal hernia which prevented the patient from walking. The pen points to the tip of the penis which is submerged into the hernia. On the left of the scrotal swelling can be seen the left testis which forms a bulge.

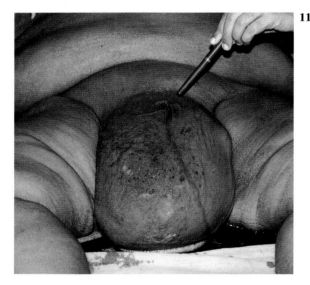

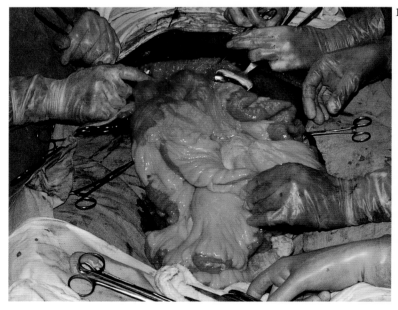

**117** The left testis (T) can be more easily seen.

**118** The hernia has been opened. It contains the whole of the small bowel, caecum, appendix, ascending colon, sigmoid colon and the omentum.

# The External Genitalia

The testicles lie in the scrotum suspended from their *spermatic cords*. Each spermatic cord with the blood supply and venous drainage of the testis contains the following.

**A** The *testicular artery*, a long branch direct from the abdominal aorta.

**B** Small arteries of the vas deferens.

**C** Cremaster branches of the inferior vesical and inferior epigastric arteries.

**D** The *testicular vein* arises from the *pampiniform plexus* of veins in and around the cord. The right enters the inferior vena cava directly. The left joins the side of the left renal vein (**119**).

**E** The *vas deferens* which feels like a piece of string, lies posteriorly in the cord and is a continuation of the 6 metre coiled canal of the epididymis. It emerges from the medial side of the tail of the epididymis at the lower posterior extremity of the testis and passes from the internal inguinal ring over the ureter in the pelvis to reach the medial extremity of the *seminal vesicle*. The vas deferens joins with the outlet of the seminal vesicle to form the *common ejaculatory duct* which opens into the prostatic urethra (**120**).

**F** The striated *cremaster muscle* derived from the internal oblique that elevates the testicle when it contracts.

At the back of the testis is attached the epididymis, shaped like a slug with a thickened head above and a more narrow tail below. Approximately 20 small ducts draining the *seminiferous tubules* of the testis – the *vasa efferentia*, pass from the upper posterior part of the testis to the head of the epididymis where they join the long coiled canal of the epididymis. The testicle has a tough fibrous coat the *tunica albuginea* and superficial to this is the *visceral tunica vaginalis*. Within the testis the germ cells divide and differentiate into mature spermatozoa, which are liberated into the seminiferous tubules (**121**, **122**). The testis is mobile within the parietal tunica vaginalis and can twist around the spermatic cord. This is an important surgical emergency, sometimes diagnosed late due to pain referred from the testicle to the lower abdomen, L1, which may fail to direct attention to the strangulating testis.

The scrotal skin has a corrugated appearance which is variable according to the tone of smooth muscle fibres of the *dartos muscle*. The two sides of the scrotum are separated from each other. A testicle may fail to descend due to arrest on its normal pathway, or it may stray away on an ectopic course, in which case by far the most common site for its malposition is above and superficial to the external inguinal ring in the superficial inguinal pouch (see **100**)

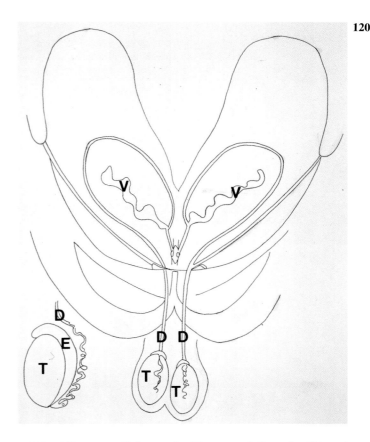

**120**

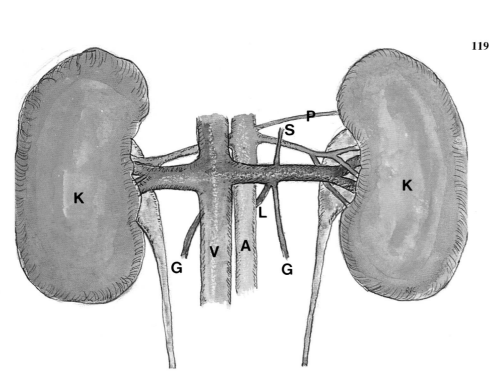

**119**

**119**  Diagram of aorta (A), vena cava (V), kidneys (K) and renal vessels. An upper polar artery (P) is shown on the left side. The gonadal vein (G) on the left enters the renal vein and on the right the vena cava. The left adrenal vein (S) joins the renal vein opposite the gonadal. A lumber vein (L) is seen curling around the arota. This vessel may be damaged during aortic aneurysm surgery.

**120**  Diagram of the testis (T), vasa deferentia (D) and seminal vesicles (V). In the lower left corner is a diagram of the relationship of the testis to the epididymis (E) and vas deferens (D) viewed from the side. The vas deferens passes through the inguinal canal and joins the seminal vesicles from where the ejaculatory duct opens beside the verumontanum in the prostatic urethra.

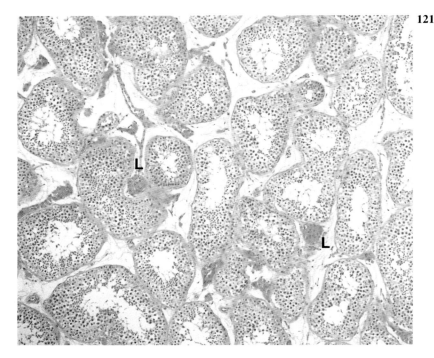

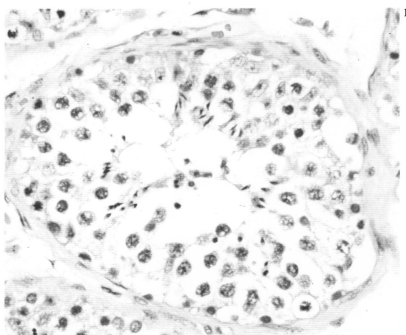

**121** Low power histology of the testis, showing the seminiferous tubules and collections of interstitial Leydig cells (L).

**122** High power histology of a seminiferous tubule. The mature spermatozoa are released into the tubular lumen.

# The Perineum

The perineum consists of an *anal triangle* posteriorly and the *urogenital triangle* in front (**123**). The anal triangle contains the anus and external sphincter, the middle portion of which loops around the anus from the *coccyx* behind to the *perineal body* in front. On each side is an *ischio-rectal fossa* lying below the pelvic diaphragm of the *levatores ani*, the lateral wall formed by the *obturator internus*, on which lies the fibrous *canal of Alcock\**. The canal contains the *pudendal vessels* and *nerves* which reach it via the *lesser sciatic foramen* from the gluteal region. They supply the anus, the external sphincter via the *inferior rectal* branches, and continue into the urogenital triangle to the external genitalia as the *dorsal nerve of the penis* and the *perineal nerve* which supplies the scrotum or labia.

The ischio-rectal fossae can become infected, usually by pyogenic organisms causing an intensely painful swelling beside the anus (**124**). This commonly bursts out through the overlying skin but can also drain into the rectum causing a chronic sinus or a fistula between the skin and the rectum. A less serious and more superficial perianal

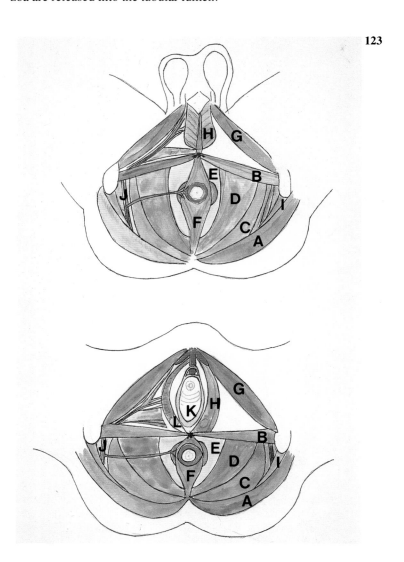

**123** Diagram of the perineum; male above, female below.
(A), gluteus maximus; (B), superficial transverse perineal muscles; (C), ischiococcygeus muscles; (D), iliococcygeus muscles; (E), puborectalis; (F), external rectal sphincter; (G), ischiocavernosus muscles; (H), bulbospongiosus muscles; (I), sacrotuberous ligament; (J) internal pudendal artery and pudendal nerve lying in Alcock's canal on the surface of the obturator internus; (K), vagina; (L), Bartholin's gland.

\* Alcock, Benjamin (1801-date of death unknown) Professor of Anatomy – Cork.

**124** CT scan showing right ischiorectal abscess which has displaced the rectum (R) to the left and caused induration of the right obturator internus muscle (i).

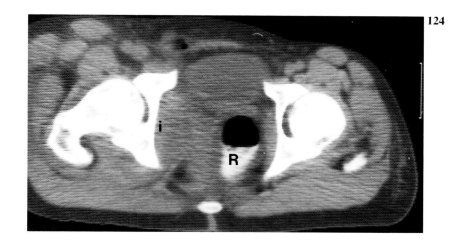

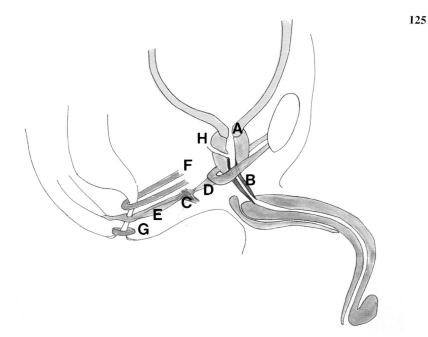

**125** Diagram of the male bladder, prostate and urethra showing the internal bladder neck urethral sphincter (A), the distal intrinsic urethral sphincter (B), the perineal body (C), into which are inserted the puboprostatic fibres of the levator ani (D) and the superficial external sphincter (E). Puborectalis portion of the levator ani (F), and subcutaneous external anal spincter (G). Ejaculatory duct (H) entering the prostatic urethra.

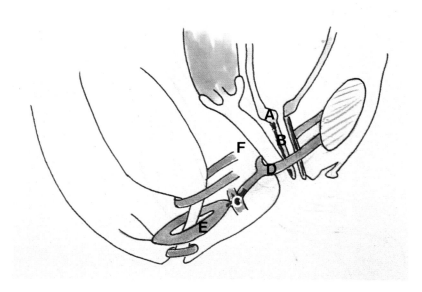

**126** In the female the arrangements are similar to the male but the intrinsic urethral external sphincter (B) extends up the whole length of the urethra to the bladder – it blends with the internal sphincter (A). The sphincter vaginae fibres are the homologue of the puboprostatic muscle (D).

abscess can also lead to sinus or fistula formation. The lymphatic drainage of the anal canal is to the *inguinal nodes*, whilst the rectum drains into the *iliac* and *preaortic nodes*. These different fields of drainage are important in the spread of cancer from these organs.

The urogenital triangle between the inferior pubic rami and a line joining the two ischial tuberosities, lies in front of the anal triangle. The *perineal membrane* is attached to the margins of the *pubic arch* and the fibromuscular perineal body which lies between the anus and the lower end of the prostate in the male, and the vagina in the female. The perineal membrane divides the urogenital triangle into *superficial* and *deep perineal pouches*. In front of it pass the *dorsal nerves* of the penis, branches of the pudendal nerves and the *dorsal vein of the penis*. Through the midline of the perineal membrane pass the urethra and the vagina in the female and on each side the internal *pudendal artery* which supplies the clitoris or in the male, the penis (**125**, **126**).

The deep perineal pouch lies between the perineal membrane and the levator ani muscles. It contains the *deep transverse perineal muscles*, the internal pudendal arteries, the dorsal nerves of the penis and the 1 cm long membranous part of the urethra, its least distensible portion. In the male two pea-sized *bulbo-urethral glands of Cowper** lie beside the urethra, their ducts pass through the perineal membrane to open into the proximal part of the *spongy urethra*. Their homologues in the female are the *greater vestibular glands of Bartholin†* which lie behind the bulb of the vestibule, superficial to the perineal membrane and open into the lower vagina posteriorly. They may become acutely inflamed.

In both sexes urinary continence depends on two sphincteric mechanisms important surgically.

**A** *Bladder neck or internal sphincter*, an extension of detrusor bladder smooth muscle around the internal urinary meatus. In the male it extends down to the midpoint of the posterior urethra where the ejaculatory ducts open on each side of a small elevation called the *verumontanum*. In the female it is less well developed. It blends with the inner smooth muscle layer of the urethra (**128, 129**). The sympathetic hypogastric plexus of nerves L1,2 stimulates the sphincter muscle and relaxes the bladder muscle, the parasympathetic pelvic splanchnic nerves stimulate the bladder muscle to contract and the sphincter to relax.

**B** *Distal* or *external urethral sphincter* forms the wall of the urethra. In the male the distal sphincter mechanisms extend from the verumontanum to the erectile tissue of the bulbar urethra, traversing the full length of the membranous urethra. In the female it extends from the bladder neck to the external urinary meatus, the whole length of the urethra. In both sexes the muscle fibres of the intramural sphincter mechanism are arranged in two layers. The outer layer is predominantly composed of 'slow twitch' striated muscle fibres which are capable of prolonged contraction and urethral occlusion: it blends with the inner layer of smooth muscle fibres. Innervation is from the pudendal and pelvic splanchnic nerves S2, 3, 4 (**128-132**).

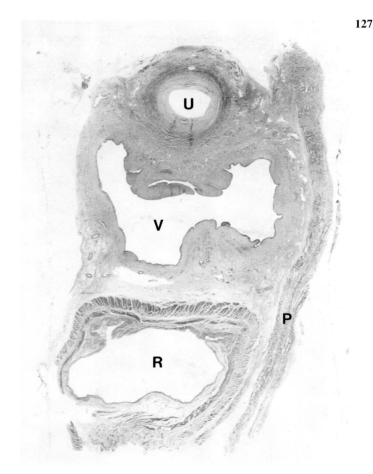

**127** Histological transverse section through female perineum at the level of the mid urethra (U), vagina (V) and rectum (R). The fibres of the pubo rectalis sling (P) are shown. Note the deficiency of muscle anterior to the urethra.

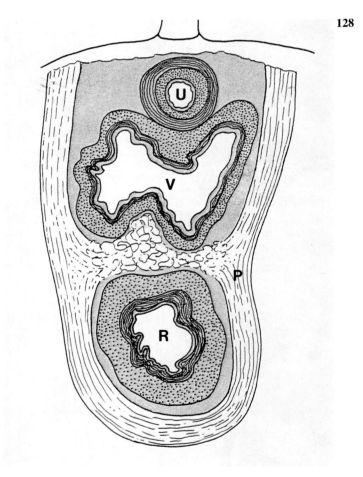

**128** Diagram of transverse section through the female perineum, labelling as for **127**.

* Cowper, William (1666-1709) London Surgeon.
† Bartholin, Caspar Secundus (1655-1738) Professor of Medicine, Anatomy and Physics, University of Copenhagen.

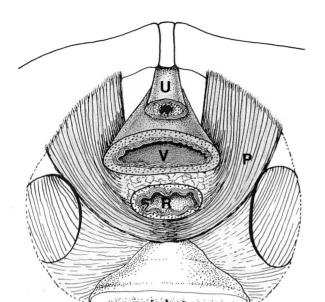

**129**

Anatomical and surgical texts commonly describe and depict an 'external' sphincter muscle mass within a 'urogenital diaphragm' encircling the membranous urethra, however, Turner-Warwick‡ has pointed out that this is fictitious and that, in the male, there is a 'pubourethral space' anterior to the urethra, between the medial margins (**132**) of the pelvic levator muscles which is of surgical importance.

**129**   Perspective diagram showing same structures as **127**.

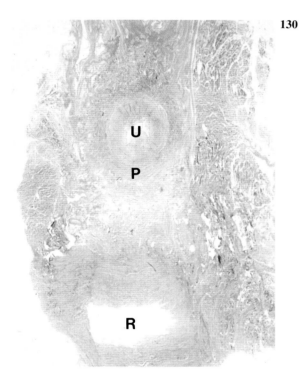

**130**

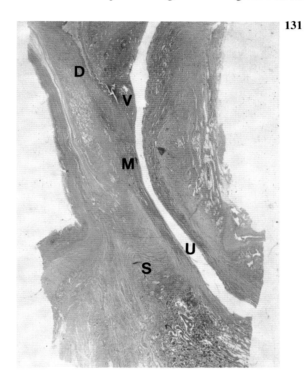

**131**

**130**   Transverse histological section of male membranous urethra showing urethra (U) with intrinsic muscle sphincter, prostate (P) and rectum (R)

**131**   Longitudinal histological section of male membranous urethra (U) showing urethral muscle (M) which inferior to the verumontanum (V) is thickened and has a striated muscle component, ejaculatory duct (D) and bulbospongiosus muscle (S).

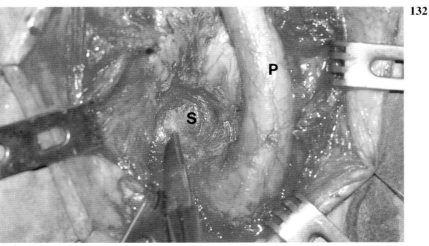

**132**

**132**   Dissection anterior to the penis (P) between it and the pubic arch. There is a space (S) with no muscle.

‡ Turner-Warwick, Richard. Contemporary Surgeon, Middlesex Hospital, London.

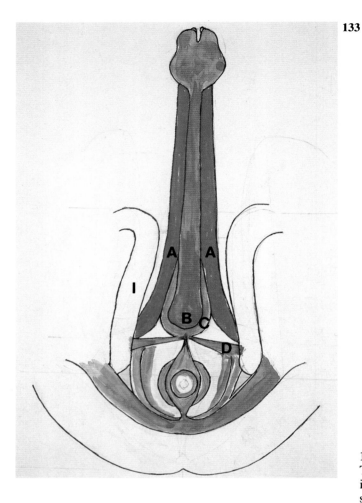

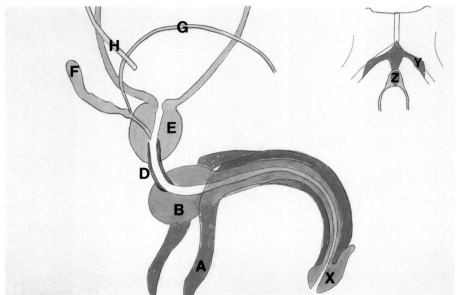

**134** Diagram of the structure of the penis showing (A) the crura which arise from the ischial rami, the corpora cavernosa, the bulb (B) through which the urethra passes as the spongy portion. The bulb becomes the corpus spongiosum, which expands at its tip as the glans penis (X). The intrinsic external urethral sphincter is shown (D), the prostate (E), the seminal vesicles (F), the vas deferens (G), ureter (H). The insert shows the clitoris which is the female homologue of the penis lying in the anterior extremity of the labia minora, which split to form the prepuce of the clitoris (P). The crura arise from the pubic arch (Y), and fuse to form the body of the clitoris and the glans at the tip (Z).

**133** Diagram of the structure of the penis showing the crura arising from the ischial rami (I). The bulb surrounded by the bulbospongiosus muscle in the midline: (A) crura, the ischiocavernosus muscles are not shown, (B) bulb, (C) bulbospongiosus muscle, (D) the superficial transverse perineal muscles.

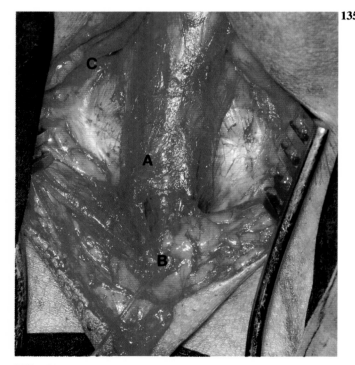

**135** Shows dissection of the bulb of the penis containing the spongy urethra. (A) the bulbospongiosus (cavernosus) muscle and (B) the perineal body posteriorly to which it is attached. (C) Ischiocavernosus muscles overlying the crura.

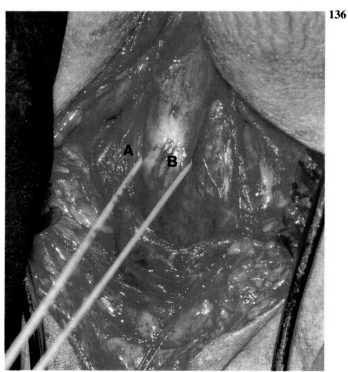

**136** On further dissection of the penis the bulbospongiosus muscle (A) has been split in the midline and separated from the bulb (B) around which has been passed a yellow sling.

Posterior to the membranous urethra in the male and to the vagina in the female, lying in front of the ano-rectal junction, there is a fibromuscular condensation called the *perineal body*. Inserted into this posteriorly is the superficial external anal sphincter and laterally are attached the *superficial* and *deep transverse perineal* muscles which arise from the ischial rami. Antero-laterally in the male, the *levator prostatae* and in the female the *pubo-vaginal* (sphincter vaginae) components of the pelvic floor levator muscles pass downwards and backwards from the lateral part of the posterior surface of the pubis and fascia overlying the obturator internis to insert into the perineal body. They form a sling around the posterior wall of the urethra and the apex of the prostate in the male, and around the vagina in the female. When these muscles contract they can close the lumen of the urethra momentarily but they are predominantly composed of 'fast' striated muscle fibres which are unable to maintain a sustained contraction and are consequently incapable of maintaining urinary continence.

The smooth muscle fibres of both the detrusor and its extension that forms the bladder neck mechanism in the female, are chiefly innervated by cholinergic nerve endings, but have in addition adrenergic fibres. The seminal vesicles and male bladder neck are similarly innervated.

During seminal emission the internal sphincter mechanism contracts preventing retrograde flow of semen into the bladder. The function of the bulbospongiosus muscle surrounding the bulbar urethra is to expel urine after voiding and to convert a seminal emission into ejaculation, aided by the turgescence of the bulbo-spongy erectile tissue.

When an enlarged prostate causes bladder outlet obstruction and has to be removed, the bladder neck sphincter mechanism is damaged; seminal fluid is retained within the prostatic cavity until it is voided with urine. Urinary continence after prostatectomy is then dependent upon the thin delicate structure of the distal sphincter mechanism which can be damaged by ignorant surgical manipulations of the urethra between the verumontanum and the bulb.

The superficial perineal pouch contains the origin of the spongy urethra, the root of the penis and the *superficial perineal muscles* – the superficial transverse perinei, the ischio-cavernosus inserted into the crus and the bulbospongiosus. Urine extravasating from a ruptured, spongy urethra, will pass into the scrotum and penis and in front of the pubis to the anterior abdominal wall.

The erectile tissue of the penis consists of two *crura* attached to the pubic arch, which become the *corpora cavernosa*, lying beside each other on the dorsum and the single *corpus spongiosum* lying ventrally, expanded as the proximal *bulb* and into the *glans* distally. The bulb lies on the perineal membrane, it is traversed by the urethra. The crura arise from the pubic arch (**133**). In the female, the bulb is divided around the vagina and the clitoris is the homologue of the penis with similar structure (**134**). The corpora cavernosa are surrounded by strong fibrous sheaths, whereas the sheath of the corpus spongiosum is less dense (**135**, **136**). All three are enclosed in the *penile fascia*. The *prepuce*, removed in the operation of circumcision, is a skin fold surrounding the glans and attached to it ventrally by the *frenulum* (**137-142**).

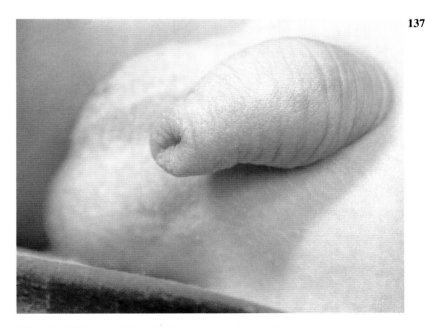

**137**  A child with phimosis for whom a circumcision was required.

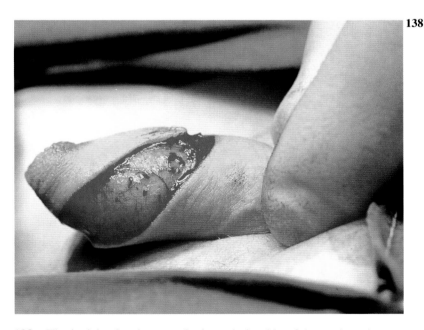

**138**  The incision has been made through the skin of the penis at the proximal level of the glans.

Erection depends on a good arterial blood supply and poorly understood autonomic nervous reflexes that block venous outflow.

The *vulva* has in front of it a pad of fat over the pubis anteriorly, the *mons veneris* behind which is the *anterior commissure* of the *labia majora*. These are lip-like skin folds which surround the pudendal cleft and unite posteriorly in front of the anus as the *posterior commissure* (**143, 144**).

The more delicate *labia minora* lie within the labia majora; they surround the vaginal vestibule and blend anteriorly with the clitoris forming its prepuce. The *urethral orifice* lies in front of the vaginal vestibule with the *vaginal introitus* behind (**145, 146**). The female urethra is 3 cm in length, it is straight and lies in the anterior vaginal wall.

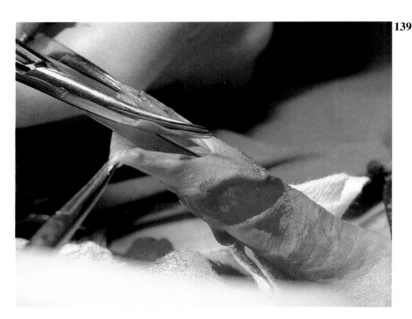

**139** The prepuce is divided.

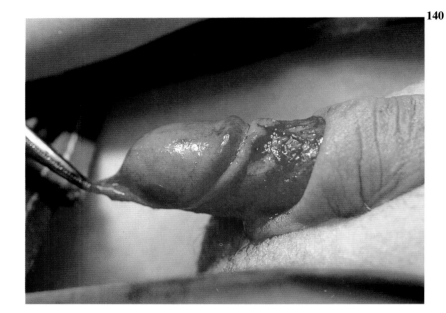

**140** The prepuce has been removed and the defect is shown.

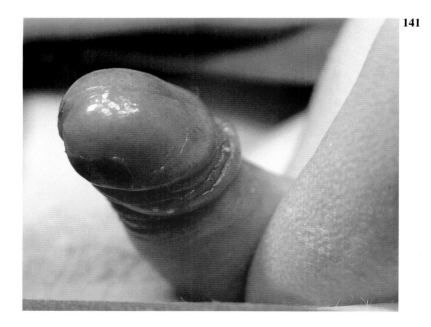

**141** The proximal and distal skin edges are brought together.

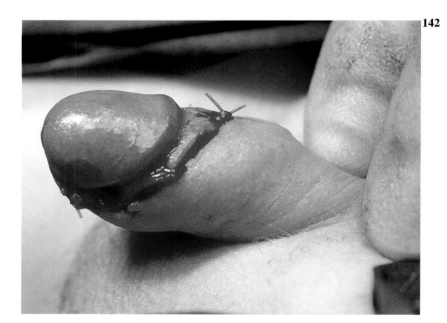

**142** The skin is closed with interrupted stitches and final suturing has been completed.

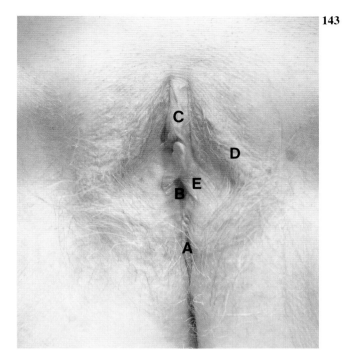

**143**   The appearance of the vulva in an elderly patient. The anus is seen posteriorly (A), the vaginal introitus (B), clitoris (C), labia majora (D), labia minora (E).

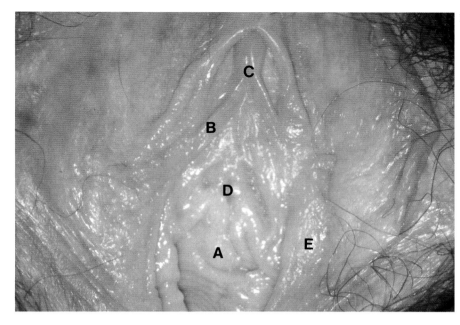

**144**   The vulva of a woman of child-bearing age with vaginal introitus (A), the labia minora (B), clitoris (C), urethra (D), labia majora (E).

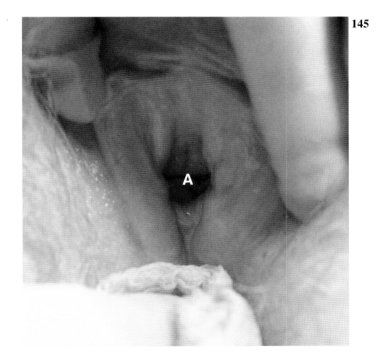

**145**   The labia minora have been separated to show the urethral orifice (A).

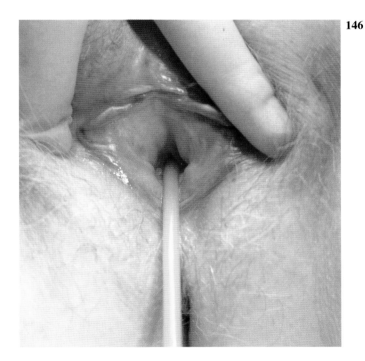

**146**   A catheter has been inserted in the urethral orifice which lies in the anterior vaginal wall and is closely applied to the wall throughout its course.

# The Diaphragm

The diaphragm is a double cupola musculo-tendinous dome, consisting of peripheral striated muscle and a forward pointing trefoil-shaped *central tendon* (**147**). It separates the chest from the abdomen. Attached to the L1, 2 and 3 vertebral bodies, the right and left crura pass on either side of the aorta, *thoracic duct* and *azygos vein* at the level of L1. They meet in front and cross, forming the *median arcuate ligament*. The right crus then passes to the left and anteriorly surrounding the oesophagus as it traverses the diaphragm at the level of T10. Lateral to the crura, the diaphragm is attached to the *medial* and *lateral arcuate ligaments*. The medial arcuate ligament passes from the body of L1 vertebrum to its transverse process over the psoas muscle. The lateral arcuate ligament arises from the transverse process of L1 and passes over the *quadratus lumborum* muscle to the 12th rib. The sympathetic chain passes under the medial arcuate ligament and the splanchnic nerves pierce the crura. The diaphragm also receives six slips from the lower six costal cartilages interdigitating with the transversus abdominis origin and two small muscle fibres come from the xiphisternum.

The inferior vena cava passes through the central tendon at the level of T9. The abdominal diaphragmatic surface is covered with peritoneum. The thoracic surface is covered with pleura laterally and is densely fused with pericardium over the central tendon. The superior surface of the liver, upper poles of the kidneys, spleen and adrenal glands are all close and important surgical anatomical

**147**

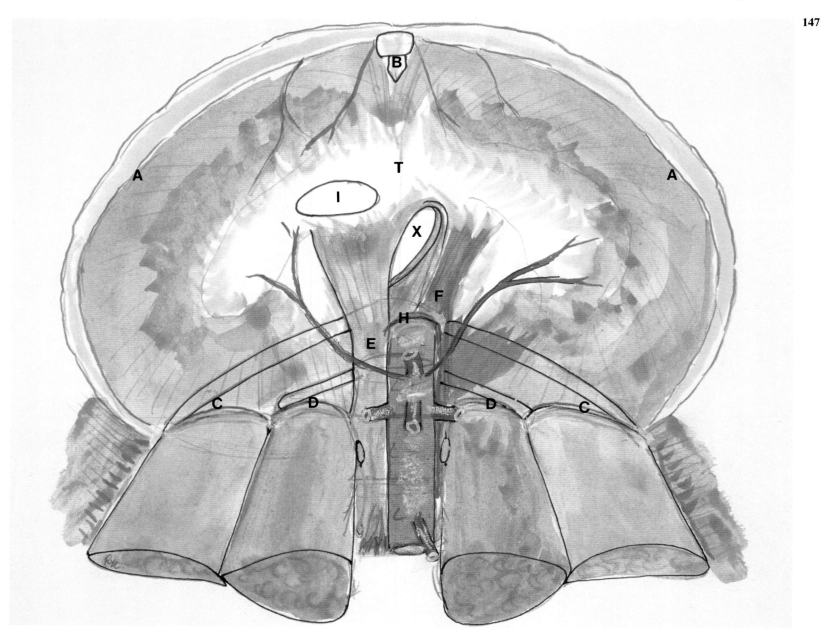

**147** Diagram of the diaphragm shows its origin from the ribs and costal cartilages (A), the xiphisternum (B), the lateral arcuate ligament overlying the quadratus lumborum (C), and the medial arcuate ligament overlying the psoas (D), the right and left crura (E) and (F). The right crus decussates to form the oesophageal hiatus at the level T10 (X). The aorta passes under the median arcuate ligament (H) at the level of T12 and the orifice for the inferior vena cava (I) is in the ventral trefoil tendon of the diaphragm (T) at the level of T9.

60

relations of the pleural cavity. The pericardium can be approached from the abdomen by incising the central tendon.

Each cupola of the diaphragm is innervated by its own phrenic nerve derived from C3, 4 and 5. The diaphragm develops in the cervical region and in its descent takes its nerves with it through the thoracic inlet and along the side of the pericardium.

Other important nerves coming through the diaphragm are:

*The vagi.* The tenth cranial nerves, which supply the upper abdominal organs, the foregut and midgut. The branches to the stomach are important surgically. Each vagus arises from the medulla and leaves the skull through the jugular foramen, passes through the neck via the thoracic inlet into the chest where lying posterior to the oesophagus the right and left vagi interconnect in the *oesphageal plexus* and pass into the abdomen usually as two nerves, a posterior vagal trunk (**148**) mainly from the right vagus and an anterior vagal trunk mainly from the left (**149**). Branches pass to the liver in the lesser omentum and also to the *sympathetic coeliac plexus* which distributes the vagus to the pancreas, spleen, kidneys, adrenals and via the superior mesenteric artery to the small bowel and large bowel as far as the splenic flexure.

The most important nerves supplying the stomach are fine filamentous branches, the *anterior* and *posterior nerves of Latarget**, which lie in the lesser omentum along the lesser curve of the stomach, giving off branches to the anterior and posterior walls of the stomach respectively (**150, 151**). The branches to the body and fundus of the stomach are secreto-motor; stimulation causes outpouring of gastric juice, high in acidity. The fibres from the termination of the nerves of Latarget to the antrum of the stomach are motor to the pylorus.

Until recently one the most popular operations for the treatment of duodenal ulcer was to cut the vagal trunks close to the oesophago-gastric junction to reduce the acid secretion of the stomach. This truncal vagotomy denervated the pylorus and led to gastric stasis, the stomach being unable to empty. To overcome this a pyloroplasty or gastrojejunostomy was necessary (**152**). Recently a highly selective

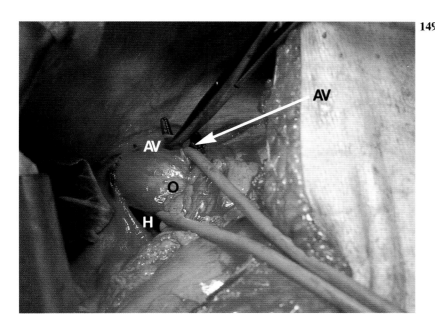

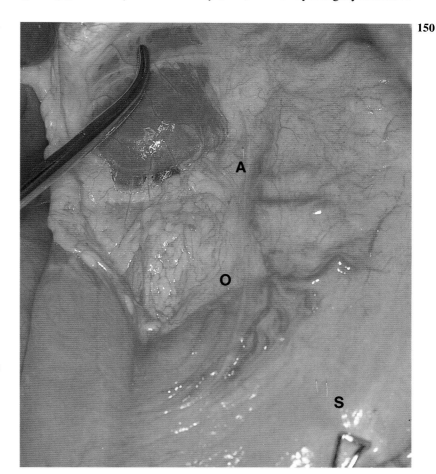

**148** The intra-abdominal oesophagus (O) is shown dissected from the oesophageal hiatus (H) in the diaphragm. The forceps hold up the posterior vagal trunk (PV).

**149** Same dissection as **148**. The forceps hold up the anterior vagal trunk (AV).

**150** Photograph of the lesser omentum (O) showing the body of the stomach to the right and below (S), the liver above and the anterior nerve of Latarget can be seen as a thin white strand (A). The forceps overlie vagal fibres passing in the lesser omentum to the liver.

*Latarget, André (1876-1947) Professor of Anatomy – Lyon.

vagotomy has been introduced in which the nerves of Latarget are most carefully preserved and the individual branches passing to the lesser curve, above and behind, are divided with the blood vessels, leaving the motor supply to the pylorus intact. This achieves the objective of cutting down the acid production by the stomach and a drainage procedure is not necessary since the pylorus can still function (**153**, **154**).

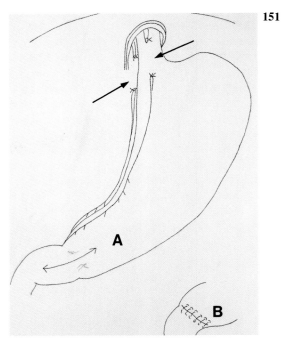

**151**

**151**  The operation of truncal vagotomy in which 2 cm of the anterior and posterior main vagal trunks are excised (arrows). Because this denervates the muscular antrum of the stomach and paralyses the opening of the pyloric sphincter it is necessary for a drainage procedure to be performed; for example a pyloroplasty shown here in which an incision is made along the arrows (A) longitudinally and closed transversely (B).

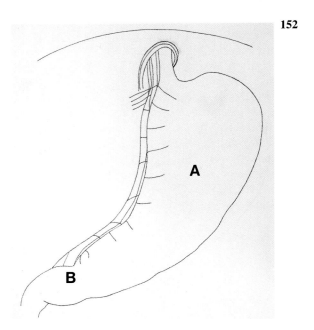

**152**

**152**  Diagram of the nerves of Latarget which are long thin filamentous structures passing from the anterior and posterior vagal trunks in the anterior and posterior lamellae of the lesser omentum. Branches are given to the body of the stomach (A), which are secretor motor. The branches to the antrum (B) supply the muscles of the antrum and allow the pyloric sphincter to open.

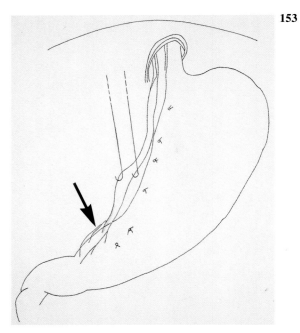

**153**

**153**  Diagram of a highly selective vagotomy in which the branches from the nerves of Latarget to the body of the stomach are ligated and divided and the supply to the antrum is kept intact (arrow).

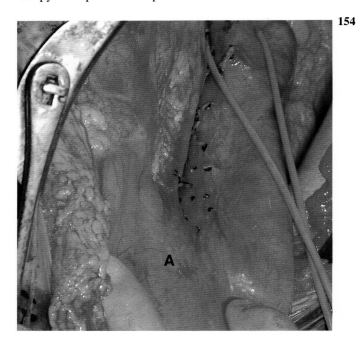

**154**

**154**  Shows the operation completed. The black ligatures show where the branches have been ligated and divided. Of necessity the blood vessels are also sacrificed in this procedure. The rubber sling surrounds the abdominal portion of the oseophagus. The antrum of the stomach (A) retains its nerve supply.

The *sympathetic nerve* supply to the foregut and midgut arises in the thoracic cord, T6-L1. The white rami join the thoracic sympathetic ganglia, from which grey rami reach the abdomen, as *greater*, *lesser* and *least splanchnic nerves* passing through the crura to form the large autonomic coeliac plexuses and smaller autonomic plexuses around all the major arteries. Strictly, the sympathetic system is an efferent system, but accompanying the sympathetic nerves are important sensory fibres, which like all other sensory fibres pass to *dorsal root ganglia*. These are responsible for transmission of visceral pain, usually due to stretch of smooth muscle, which is interpreted as referred pain to the corresponding segmental somatic sensory area. (See page 121).

*The quadratus lumborum* passes from the 12th rib to the iliac crest. Medial to it posteriorly lies the lumbar spine and the powerful erector spinae muscles behind the vertebral transverse processes and between them and the vertebral spines, supplied by the posterior primary rami of segmental nerves.

*Psoas major.* In front of the lumbar tranverse processes, between them and the vertebral bodies, the psoas major muscles arise and pass into the pelvis, the tendons lying in front of the hip joint *en route* for insertion to the femoral *lesser trochanter*. Psoas contraction stabilises the lumbar spine and flexes and internally rotates the hip. The nerves are supplied by anterior primary rami of segmental nerves from the lumbar nerve plexus, which is formed within the muscle substance. The plexus supplies the lower limbs.

*The iliacus muscle* arises from the inner curved surface of the ileum in the false pelvis. It passes lateral to the psoas and joins its tendon.

*The lumbar and sacral nerve plexus* (**155**, **156**). The genito-femoral nerve, L1, 2 emerges from the front of the upper surface of psoas major muscle, down which it runs to give a genital branch to the cremaster muscle and scrotum and a femoral branch, sensory to the upper part of the thigh just below the inguinal ligament. The *femoral*

**155**

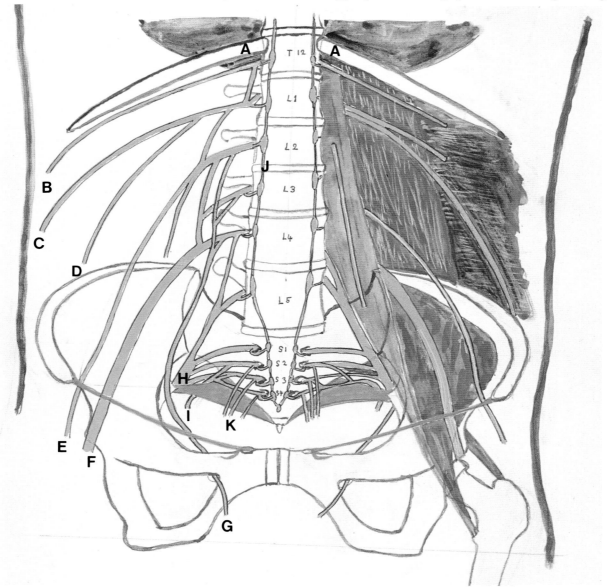

**155** Diagram of the lumbo-sacral plexus of nerves, showing the segmental arrangement of the main nerves on the right and their main relationship to the muscles of the abdomen and pelvis on the left. The pleura is indicated behind the upper part of the 12th ribs (A). The subcostal nerve (B), ilio-inguinal and ilio-epigastric (C) and (D). The lateral cutaneous nerve of the thigh (E), femoral nerve (F), the obturator nerve (G), the sciatic nerve (H), the pudendal nerve (I), the lumbar sympathetic chain (J), the pelvic splanchnic nervi erigentes (K).

and *obturator* nerves (L 2, 3, 4) arise from the lumbar plexus, which is formed within the psoas muscle from the anterior primary rami of L1-5. The femoral nerve lies between the psoas and iliacus muscles and passes over the hip joint into the femoral triangle, lateral to the femoral artery, beneath the inguinal ligament. The obturator nerve is formed medial to the psoas and passes underneath the ovary through the upper part of the obturator foramen to supply the hip adductors and the *obturator externus* which externally rotates the hip (**157**). Ovarian disease will often give rise to pain referred to the upper medial thigh because of the close relationship of the ovary to the obturator nerve.

*The sacral plexus* (L4, 5 and S1, 2, 3, 4) lies on the *piriformis muscle* where it arises from the front of the sacrum *en route* to the greater sciatic foramen. The largest branch of the sacral plexus is the *sciatic nerve*, which passes into the *gluteal* region through the greater sciatic foramen to the back of the thigh. Other important branches are the gluteal and pudendal nerves.

*Autonomic nerves of the pelvis.* In front of the sacrum lie the sacral parasympathetic *pelvic splanchnic nerves* (S2, 3 and 4), whilst just above and in front of the body of L5 is the *sympathetic hypogastric plexus* of *presacral nerves*. The pelvic splanchnic *nervi erigentes* are

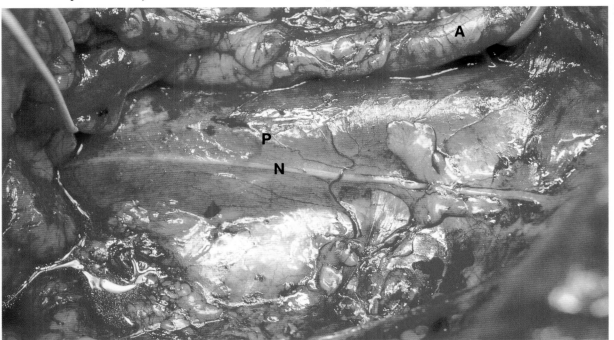

**156**

**156**   The right psoas muscle (P) showing the genito-femoral nerve (N), L1-2 lying on the front of the muscle. In the upper right hand corner a sling is passed around the right common iliac artery (A).

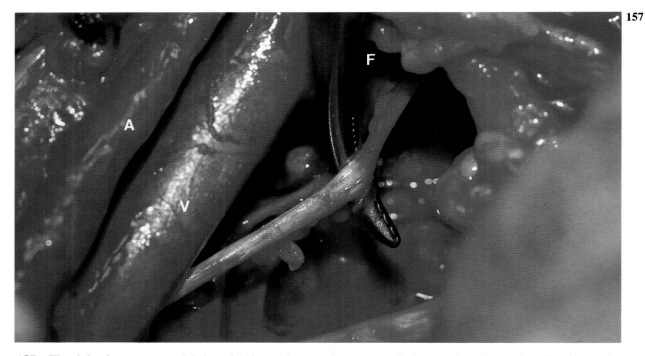

**157**

**157**   The right obturator nerve L2,3, and 4 viewed from above and laterally looking into the pelvis. It lies deep to the external iliac artery (A) and vein (V) *en route* to the upper portion of the obturator foramen (F).

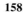

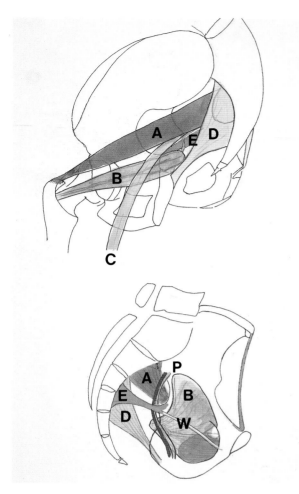

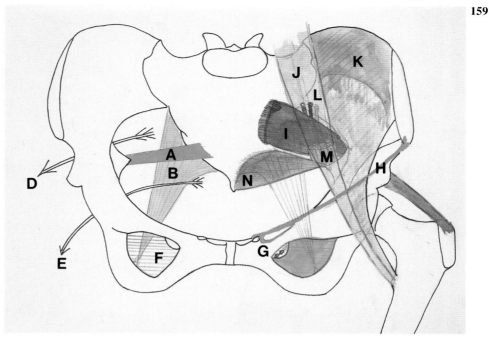

**159**  Diagram of the pelvis to show the arrangements of the main pelvic ligaments, the sacrospinous (A), sacrotuberous (B) providing the outlets of the greater and lesser sciatic foramina (D) and (E), obturator membrane (F), the obturator foramen through which the obturator vessels pass (G), the inguinal ligament (H), the piriformis muscle (I), the psoas muscle (J), the iliacus muscle (K), the superior gluteal vessels (L), the sciatic nerve (M), the coccygeus muscle (N).

**158**  Diagram of the pelvis. Oblique view above, lateral view of the hemi-pelvis below. In the upper diagram the piriformis muscle is shown (A), the obturator internis coming through the lesser sciatic foramen (B), the sciatic nerve (C), coming through the greater sciatic foramen, the sacrotuberous ligament (D), the sacrospinous ligament (E). The white line (W) from which the levator ani muscle arises is indicated in the lower diagram overlying the obturator internus (P). The internal pudendal artery and the pudendal nerve are shown passing out of the pelvis, via the greater sciatic foramen and then immediately into the pelvis again through the lesser sciatic notch, to lie in Alcock's canal on the lateral wall of the ishio-rectal fossa.

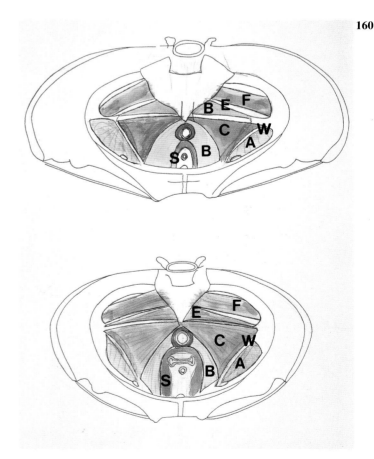

**160**  Diagram of the pelvic diaphragm from above; male upper diagram, female lower diagram. The obturator internus muscle (A), the white line (W) from which arise the pubo-coccygeus (B), and ilio-coccygeus (C), both parts of the levator ani. The coccygeus (E), and the piriformis (F) are posterior. The levator prostatae in the male and sphincter vaginae in the female (S). The pubo-rectalis is part of the pubo-coccygeus forming a U-shaped sling around the rectum.

responsible for the erection of the penis and clitoris. The hypo-gastric sympathetic nerves (white rami from T12 and L1) control ejaculation in the male. Sensory nerves in the skin of the genitalia, sensory nerves travelling with the autonomic nerves, spinal ascending and descending tracts and centres in the hind, mid and forebrain, all play a part in the complicated motor functions of mating.

*The diaphragm of the pelvic floor.* In the wall of the true pelvis, arising from the *obturator membrane*, the margins of the obturator foramen and bone behind it, lies the *obturator internus* muscle which passes out of the pelvis via the lesser sciatic foramen. This is a key anatomical muscle, whose strange course is related to many important structures (**158**). The integrity of the pelvic outlet is maintained by a combination of muscles, the pelvic diaphragm, formed on each side by the *coccygeus* and the levator ani, which is really two muscles the *ilio-*and *pubo-coccygeus*. These striated muscles are unusual in maintaining a constant involuntary tonus. The coccygeus arises from the *ischial spine* and passes fan shaped to the coccyx and sacrum. It lies on the upper pelvic surface of the *sacrospinous ligament* (**159**).

The ilio-coccygeus arises from the ischial spine and parietal pelvic fascia over the posterior part of the obturator internus where the fascia forms a thickened white line and is inserted into the coccyx and the median raphe extending to the anal canal. The pubo-coccygeus arises from the back of the pubis and parietal pelvic fascia over the anterior part of the obturator internus where the white line continues. Some fibres surround the prostate in the male, as the *levator prostatae*, and the vagina in the female, as the *sphincter vaginae*. It joins the perineal body and encircles the anorectal junction, this part being called the *puborectalis*. The supporting fibres surrounding the midline structures form a series of U-shaped slings, the limbs of the 'U' attached anteriorly (**160-164**). The muscle is supplied by the perineal branch of S4 and the pudendal nerve S2, 3 and 4 from the sacral plexus. The pudendal nerve and accompanying artery and vein from the internal iliac vessels pass below the piriformis muscle through the greater sciatic foramen into the gluteal region and then across the sacrospinous ligament to reach the ischiorectal fossa via the lesser sciatic foramen (see **158**, **159**).

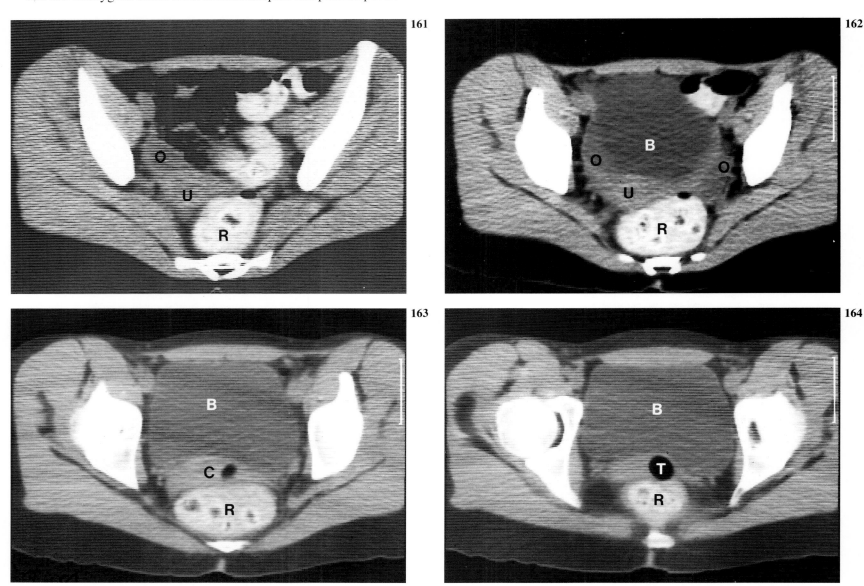

**161-164**    A series of CT images through a normal female pelvis, showing the relationships of the bladder (B), rectum (R), body of the uterus (U) and ovaries (O). On the more caudal cuts the cervix (C) is seen and the vagina is localised by the presence of air within the tampon (T).

# 3 The Organs Draining in to the Portal Vein and the Liver

The abdominal aorta, lying in front of the lumbar vertebral bodies to the left of the midline, gives off ventral and lateral visceral and symmetrical posterior *lumbar* segmental branches before it divides into the common iliac vessels in front of the body of L4.

## The Ventral Visceral Branches of the Abdominal Aorta and the Organs they Supply

**A**  *The coeliac artery* (**165-168**) arises from the aorta 4 cm below the diaphragm. There is a dense leash of nerve tissues around the coeliac artery and the adjacent aorta passing to and from the semi-lunar shaped, *coeliac sympathetic ganglia*, which constitute the coeliac plexus. This is primarily a sympathetic plexus, but it has parasympathetic contributions from the vagus nerve. Nerve fibres of the coeliac plexus are distributed to all the branches of the coeliac artery around each of which there are subsidiary autonomic nerve plexuses. There are two small lateral *phrenic* branches of the coeliac trunk at its origin or from the adjacent aorta, which supply the crura of the diaphragm, and contribute to the supply to the adrenals (see below).

The coeliac artery passes downwards and forwards to the upper surface of the pancreas where it trifurcates into left gastric, common hepatic and splenic arteries. The uppermost branch is the *left gastric* supplying the *lesser curve* of the stomach. The next and largest branch of the coeliac is the *common hepatic*, which swings forward in a curve to the right, reaching the free edge of the lesser omentum. The *right gastric*, a small vessel, usually arises directly from the common hepatic to reach the pyloric antrum or it may be a branch of the *gastroduodenal*, a substantial vessel that passes vertically down behind the duodenum, where it supplies the head of the pancreas and the *greater curve* of the stomach as the *superior pancreaticoduodenal*, and *right gastroepiploic* vessels. The superior pancreaticoduodenal anastomoses with branches of the *inferior pancreaticoduodenal* from the *superior mesenteric*. The right gastroepiploic

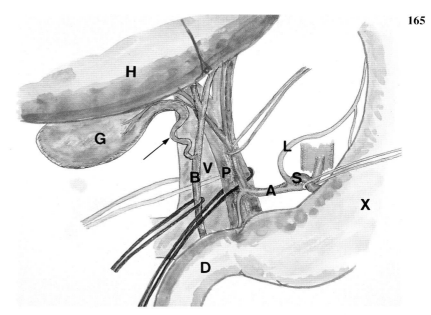

**165**

**165**  Diagram of the structures of the free edge of the lesser omentum in relation to the liver (H) duodenum (D) and vena cava (V). Gall bladder (G), cystic duct (arrow), common bile duct (B), portal vein (P), common hepatic artery (A), left gastric artery (L), splenic artery (S), stomach (X).

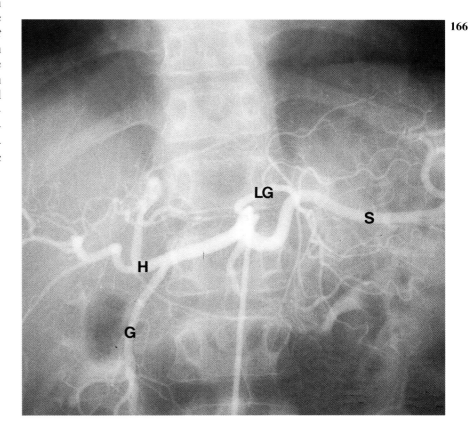

**166**

**166**  Coeliac axis arteriogram showing the splenic (S), hepatic (H), left gastric (LG) and gastro-duodenal (G) arteries.

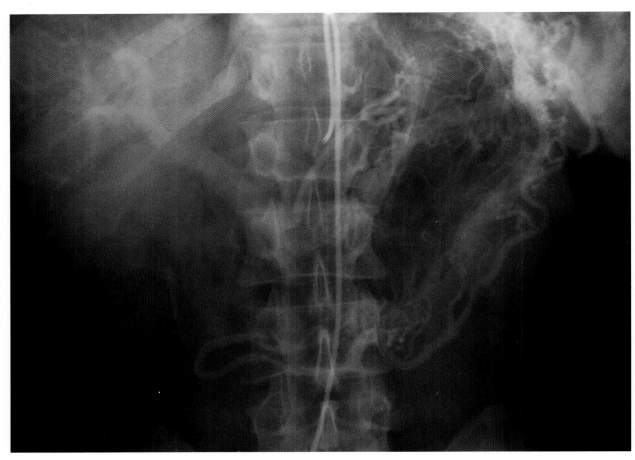

**167** Venous phase of coeliac axis arteriogram showing the gastric vein along the greater curve, and the splenic vein feeding into the portal vein.

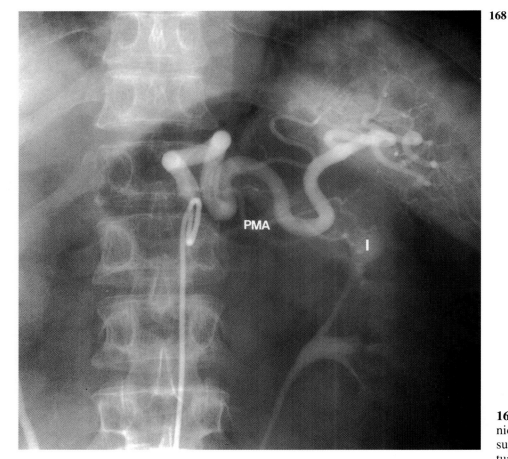

PMA

I

**168** Selective splenic arteriogram showing tortuosity of the splenic artery. The pancreatica magna artery (PMA) is demonstrated supplying the body and tail of the pancreas and insulin producing tumour (I).

forms an arcade around the greater curve of the stomach which it supplies and then joins the *left gastro-epiploic*, a branch of the *splenic*. The common hepatic then continues into the lesser omentum, to the left of the common bile duct and in front of the portal vein. It divides into the right and left hepatic arteries supplying the right and left lobes of the liver respectively. The right branch gives off the *cystic artery* which usually passes behind, but sometimes in front of the common hepatic duct to supply the gall bladder.

The third branch of the coeliac, the splenic, passes off to the left. It has an undulating course and lies above the splenic vein. It supplies the body of the pancreas and then gives off the left gastroepiploic branch which completes the arcade along the greater curvature of the stomach. The splenic artery continues towards the hilum of the spleen giving off 5-6 *short gastric arteries* which pass to the stomach. It then divides in the hilum of the spleen.

**B**  *The superior mesenteric artery* (**169**) arises 1-2 cm below the coeliac artery. It is a large vessel which passes forwards and downwards behind the neck of the pancreas and emerges between the uncinate process and the neck of the pancreas. The superior mesenteric vein lies alongside, slightly in front and to the right of the artery. Just above the origin of the artery the splenic vein joins the superior mesenteric vein to form the portal vein (**170, 171**). The superior

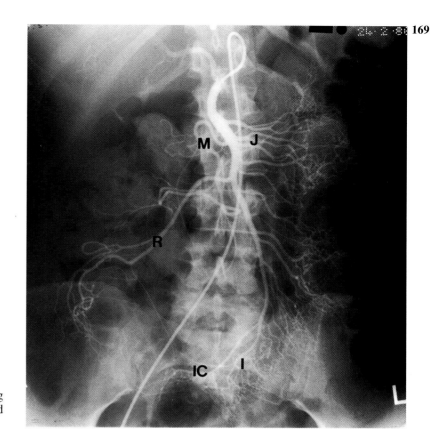

**169**  Selective superior mesenteric arteriogram showing jejunal branches (J), ileal branches (I), ileocolic (IC) and middle (M) and right (R) colic branches.

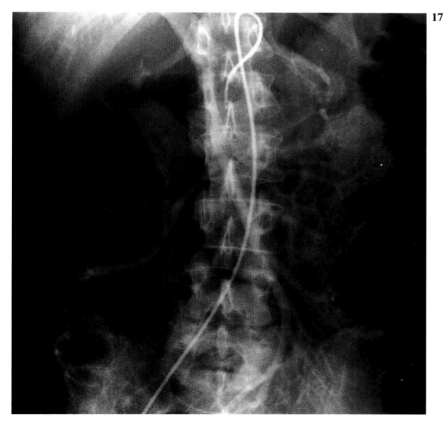

**170**  Venous phase, showing the superior mesenteric vein entering the portal vein.

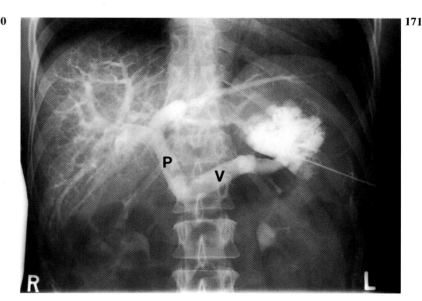

**171**  Puncture of the spleen with injection of contrast, showing the splenic vein (V) joining the superior mesenteric to form the portal vein (P).

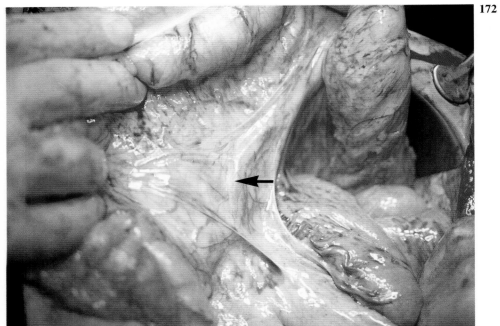

**172** The tranverse colon has been lifted up to show the transverse mesocolon containing the middle colic arterial branch of the superior mesenteric artery (arrow).

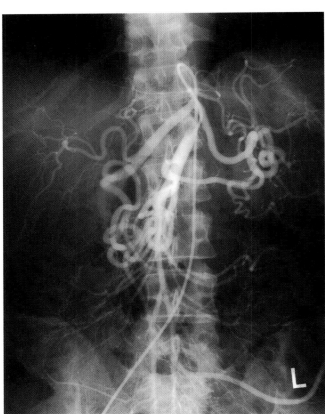

**173** Selective superior mesenteric artery injection in a case where there is blockage of both the coeliac axis and inferior mesenteric arteries with filling of the inferior mesenteric artery by an extremely enlarged collateral connection to the artery of Drummond.

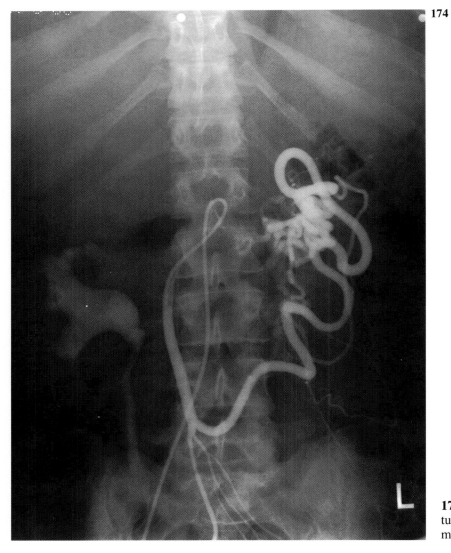

**174** Selective inferior mesenteric arteriogram in a case of a huge vascular tumour of the liver. Large collateral vessel from the inferior to the superior mesenteric artery and then to the liver.

mesenteric artery gives off the inferior pancreatico-duodenal branch and the large *middle colic*, which passes in the transverse mesocolon to supply the transverse colon (**172**). It then passes in the root of the small bowel mesentery giving off jejunal and ileal branches which form single arcades in the upper jejunum, double arcades in the lower jejunum and three or four layers of arcades in the ileum. The vessel ends as the *ileocolic artery*, giving off an *appendicular* vessel which passes in a little mesentery, to supply the appendix. The ileocolic breaks up into branches which supply the caecum and ascending colon. An anastomotic branch lies alongside the colonic wall which is fed successively by each of the colic vessels. This *marginal artery of Drummond** is important, maintaining the vascularity of colonic cut ends when these are anastomosed together (**173, 174**).

**C** *The inferior mesenteric artery* (**175**). In the middle of the course of the abdominal aorta, some 5-6 cm proximal to its bifurcation, the inferior mesenteric arises and passes downwards, forwards and to the left to enter the pelvic mesocolon. A variable number of *left colic* branches are given off, which anastomose with branches of the middle colic (superior mesenteric) and with each other via the marginal artery. Three or four sigmoid branches pass in the pelvic mesocolon to supply the sigmoid colon. The inferior mesenteric ends as the superior rectal which is the main supply of the rectum down to the ano-rectal junction. It anastomoses with branches of the middle rectal arteries (small branches of the internal iliac arteries) and the inferior rectal arterial branches of the internal pudendal which supply the anal canal. The inferior mesenteric vein receives branches corresponding to the arteries, it lies on the left side of the artery and passes up behind the pancreas to join the splenic vein (**176**).

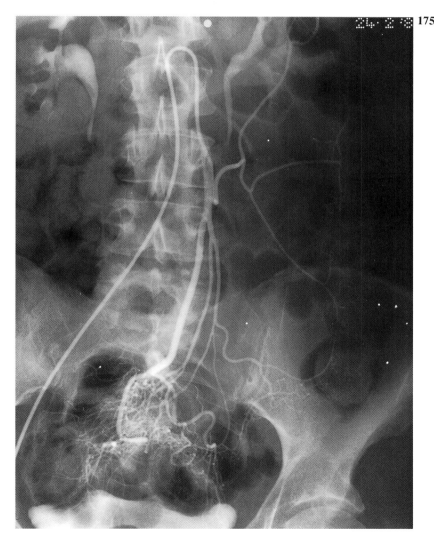

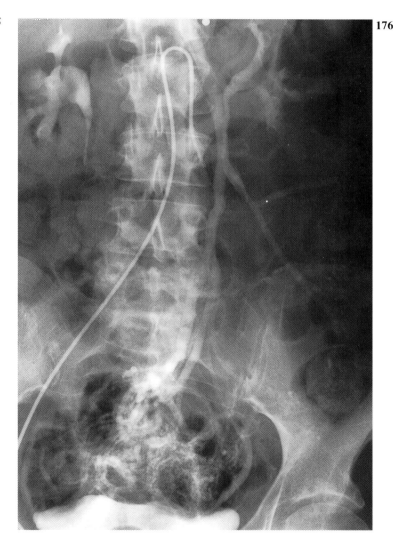

**175**  Selective inferior mesenteric arteriogram showing the superior left colic, inferior left colic and superior rectal arteries.

**176**  Venous phase of inferior mesenteric arteriogram.

*Drummond, Hamilton (1852-1932) Newcastle Surgeon.

71

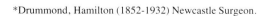

# Abdominal Oesophagus and Stomach

Their topography has been outlined (Chapter 1). The thoracic portion

**A** The muscle fibres of the right crus of the diaphragm (**179**).
**B** The angle of entry into the stomach discourages reflux – the angle of His*.

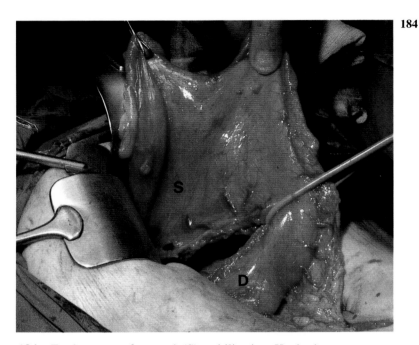

**184** Further stage of stomach (S) mobilization. Kocher's manoeuvre has been performed. Duodenum (D).

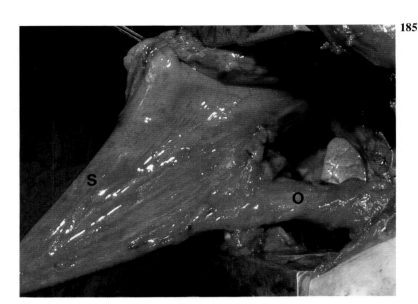

**185** Viewed through the left side of the chest, the stomach (S) has been brought up into the chest with the right gastric and the right gastro-epiploic arteries being the only remaining blood vessels. Oesophagus (O).

## The Duodenum

The duodenum begins immediately distal to the pyloric sphincter of intrinsic gastric muscle (**186**). The junction is marked by a small prepyloric vein of Mayo* (**187**). The duodenum is 20 cm long, is a retroperitoneal C-shaped portion of the small bowel, the concavity of the C pointing to the left (**188**). It receives the joint entry of the main *pancreatic* and *common bile ducts* into the *ampulla of Vater†*, which is protected by the important *sphincter of Oddi‡*, a condensation of

duodenal wall muscle. The first part of the duodenum is 2.5 cm long (**189**). It is the chief site of duodenal ulceration, with its complications of perforation (anterior), haemorrhage (posterior into the head of the pancreas) and stenosis caused by chronic fibrosis and shrinkage of scar tissue. The second part descends vertically for 5 cm and receives the ampulla of Vater (**190, 191**). It is related laterally to the

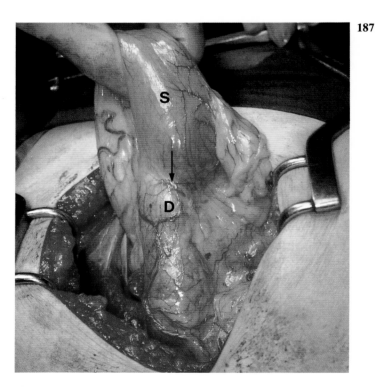

**187** The gastro-duodenal junction is marked externally by the prepyloric vein of Mayo (arrow). Stomach (S), duodenum (D).

**186** Histology of the gastro-duodenal junction. There is considerable smooth muscle mass in the lower right corner, which is the pyloric sphincter (P). The gastric mucosa (G) in the upper right corner changes to duodenal mucosa (D) on the left with Brunners glands (B) in the submucosa.

*Mayo, Charles Horace (1865-1939) and William James (1861-1939). Brothers who founded the Mayo Clinic, Rochester, Minnesota.
†Vater, Abraham (1684-1751) Professor of Anatomy – Wittenberg.
‡Oddi, Ruggero (1845-1906) Surgeon and anatomist – Rome.

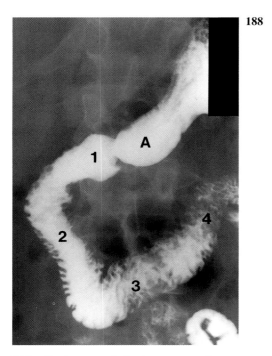

**188** Barium meal single contrast showing the pyloric antrum (A) and all four parts of the duodenum (1-4).

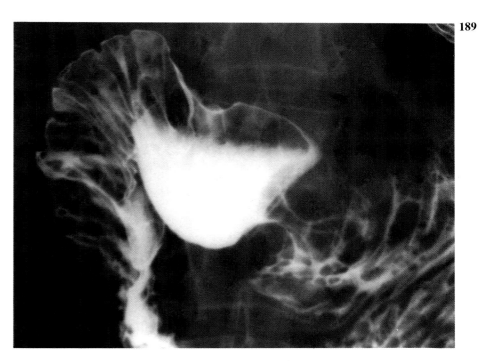

**189** Barium meal demonstrating a normal duodenal cap which has a triangular shape (the first part of the duodenum).

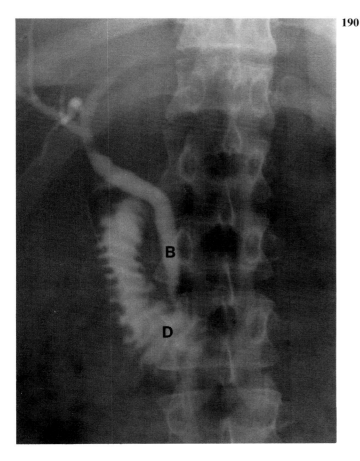

**190** An operative cholangiogram. Contrast has been passed through the cystic duct after the gall bladder has been removed. The common bile duct (B) is seen entering the duodenum (D) and the main intra-hepatic bile ducts have also been opacified.

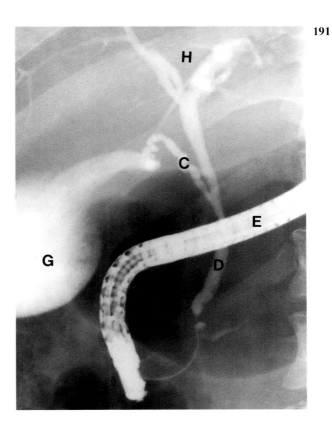

**191** An endoscopic cholangiogram – the endoscope (E) passes through the mouth to the duodenum. Via the endoscope a catheter is passed through the sphincter of Oddi. Contrast injection demonstrates the common bile duct (D) and the beaded appearance of the cystic duct (C); the gall bladder (G) is seen on the left and the branches of the common hepatic duct (H) are shown above on the right (abnormal).

hilum of the right kidney. The third part, 5 cm long, crosses the abdominal aorta below the origin of the superior mesenteric artery which in turn crosses it (**34**, page 20). The fourth part turns up towards the front held by a short fold of peritoneum within which is a smooth muscle strand extending from the right diaphragmatic crus in front of the aorta to blend with the duodenal wall – the *ligament of Treitz* – the duodenum here acquires a mesentery and becomes intraperitoneal and joins the jejunum. The duodenum receives its blood supply from the superior and inferior pancreatico-duodenal arterial branches of the coeliac and superior mesenteric arteries.

# The Small Intestine

The small intestine is a muscular tube with an inner circular smooth muscle layer and an outer longitudinal muscle layer. Its contents are normally fluid. It is approximately 6 metres long, the first 4 metres are called the *jejunum*, which is the main site of nutritional absorption. The mucosa can be felt separate from the muscular layer when the jejunal wall is rolled between the thumb and fingers, in contrast to the ileum where the wall feels as if it is all one layer. The jejunum has an excellent blood supply from the superior mesenteric artery (**192**). The remaining 2 metres of small bowel called the *ileum* resemble the jejunum, but the mesentery has a wider origin on the bowel so that fat in the mesentery tends to encroach on the bowel wall. Its main function is to absorb water from the intestinal contents.

The mucosa of the small intestine forms finger-like projections, called villi, lined by columnar epithelium. In the centre of each villus is a blind opening lymphatic channel called the *lacteal*, into which are absorbed undigested fats (**193**, **194**). There are condensations of lymphoid tissue in the bowel wall, and those in the ileum are arranged as oval plaques called Peyer's* patches, which are involved in typhoid fever. Macroscopically, the mucosa is arranged in concentric rings, the *plicae circumventes*, which help differentiate dilated small from large bowel on plain X-rays. The root of the mesentery runs from the ligament of Treitz on the left of the body of L1 to the right sacroiliac joint (**38**, page 22).

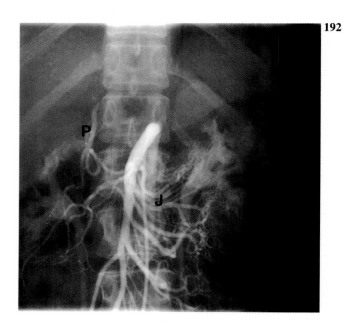

**192** Selective mesenteric arteriogram showing the branches of the jejunum (J) and the inferior pancreatico-duodenal artery (P).

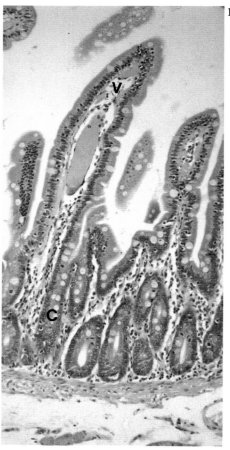

**193** Microscopy of the jejunal mucosa showing villi (V) and crypts (C) lined by columnar epithelium.

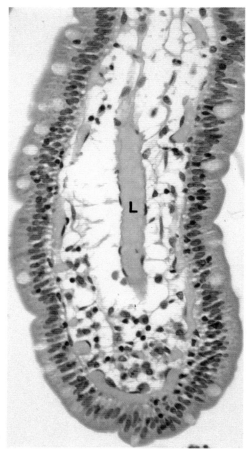

**194** High power of the villus with a central lacteal (L).

*Peyer, Johann Conrad (1653-1712) Professor of Logic, Rhetoric and Medicine – Schaff Hausen, Switzerland.

# The Appendix

The appendix is a narrow blind ending muscular tube with much lymphoid tissue in the submucosal layers, so that it resembles tonsil histology (**195, 196**). The mucosa is colonic in type. The appendicular artery is a branch of the ileocolic, a continuation of the superior mesenteric. It reaches the appendix in a small mesentery, the mesoappendix. Between this and the terminal ileum is a fold of peritoneum called the "bloodless fold of Treves†". Despite its name, it usually contains a small blood vessel that can be seen without difficulty (**197**).

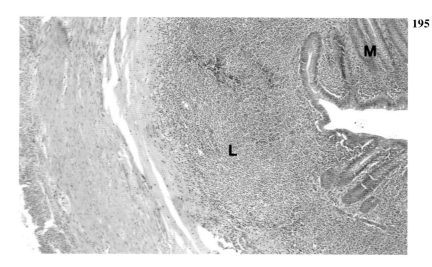

**195** Histology of the appendix. Mucosa (M) consists of straight tubular glands lined by absorptive columnar cells and goblet cells. The submucosa contains a large amount of lymphoid tissue (L).

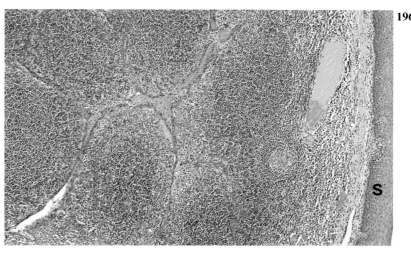

**196** Tonsil with similar condensation of lymphoid tissue. The lining is stratified squamous epithelium (S), seen on the right.

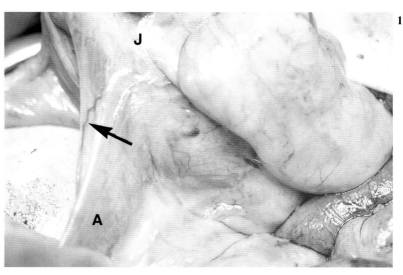

**197** The peritoneal fold from the ileo-caecal junction (J) to the base of the appendix (A), named the bloodless fold of Treves, but containing an obvious small blood vessel (arrow).

†Treves, Sir Frederick (1853-1923) Surgeon to the London Hospital.

# The Large Bowel

The large bowel absorbs water from the bowel contents and stores and evacuates the remaining faeces. The muscular wall is curiously constructed with a main circular structure and three longitudinal condensations equidistant from each other around the wall. They were thought to resemble tapeworms and are called *taeniae coli*. The blood supply of the proximal large bowel as far as the splenic flexure is from the superior mesenteric and that of the descending colon and the rest of the upper rectum is from the inferior mesenteric. The wall of the large bowel is arranged in sac-like segments called haustrations. The middle rectal arteries, branches of the anterior division of the internal iliac, supply the middle and lower rectum and anastomoses with the inferior mesenteric branch above and the inferior rectal branches of the pudendal artery supplying the anal canal below. The rectum is an extremely distensible part of the large bowel (**198**). The anal canal, 3 cm long, passes posteriorly and down from the rectum at the level of the pubo-rectalis muscle to open on the skin and is lined in its lowermost part with squamous epithelium. The junction of squamous and columnar epithelium forms the white line of Hilton.* At this level the longitudinal muscle of the rectum ceases, above it is the internal sphincter and below it the external sphincter.

The mucosa of the anal canal above Hilton's white line has an interlinking series of ridges convex inferiorly called the *dentate* ring of *anal valves*, which have no functional value. They lead above to longitudinal *anal columns* which are also mucosal ridges (**199**). The sensory nerves of the anal canal below Hilton's line are somatic from the pudendal conferring a sensitivity equivalent to that of skin to pain. Thus anal fissures are extremely painful, while ulcerating lesions in the rectum with visceral sensation are not. The lymphatics draining the lower anal canal join the inguinal nodes. The anal sphincter is very important and complicated, with both sensory and neuromotor muscular components. The two muscular sphincters are internal, smooth muscle and external, striated muscle, they overlap in the middle third of the anal canal.

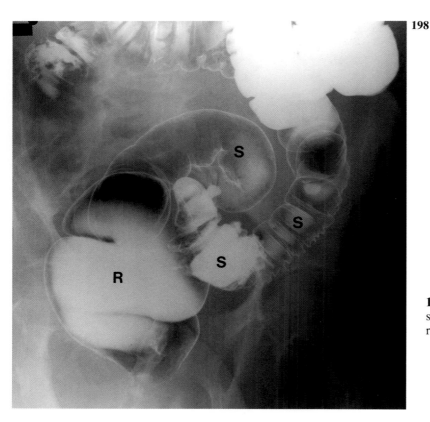

**198**　Barium enema showing the distensible rectum (R) leading to the narrower sigmoid colon (S) on the upper part of the X-ray.

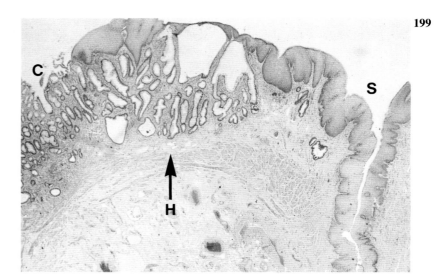

**199**　The ano-rectal junction and the white line of Hilton (H, arrowed). Right: stratified squamous epithelium (S) of the anus, left: columnar epithelium of the rectum (C).

*Hilton, John (1805-1878) Surgeon, Guys Hospital – London.

*The internal sphincter* is a condensation of the inner circular smooth muscle of the large bowel. It occupies the upper two thirds of the anal canal. Sympathetic stimulation causes it to contract and parasympathetic nerve impulses cause relaxation, similar to the internal sphincter of the bladder. There is an overriding voluntary control that will not ensure continence without help from the external sphincter. Its autonomic innervation comes from the pelvic plexus.

*The external sphincter* (**200**) has three components of striated muscle innervated by the inferior rectal branch of the pudendal nerve (S3, 4) and the perineal branch of S4.

**A** *The subcutaneous anal sphincter* is a thick ring of striated muscle which lies just deep to the involuntary *corrugator cutis ani muscle* part of the *panniculus carnosis*\*; when it contracts it causes the anal skin to draw together as if pulled by a purse string. Deep to the subcutaneous anal sphincter is a layer of fascia which passes from the outer longitudinal muscle layer of the anus at Hilton's line, laterally to the pudendal canal of Alcock, on the surface of the obturator internus. This fascia separates the deep ischio-rectal fossa from the superficial peri-anal space, in which lies the subcutaneous sphincter.

**B** *The superficial external sphincter* passes from the coccyx behind, surrounding the anus to join the perineal body in front.

**C** *The deep external anal sphincter* is a ring of striated muscle surrounding the lower part of the internal sphincter and joining the pubo-rectalis muscle posteriorly at the ano-rectal junction, where the anus is inclined backwards from the rectum. It is the most important element of the anal sphincteric mechanism in maintaining faecal continence.

The veins and lymphatics of the abdominal viscera tend to follow the arteries. The *inferior mesenteric vein* lies to the left of the artery and passes laterally in the retroperitoneal space to enter the splenic vein which it joins at right angles behind the pancreas. The superior mesenteric vein lies to the right of the artery, receiving the middle colic at the base of the mesocolon. The splenic vein enters it at right angles, the conjoined trunk forming the portal vein, which passes behind the common bile duct and the hepatic artery in the free edge of the lesser omentum. Most of the veins of the stomach drain into the splenic vein. The large left gastric or coronary vein usually joins the splenic but may open into the portal directly.

**200**

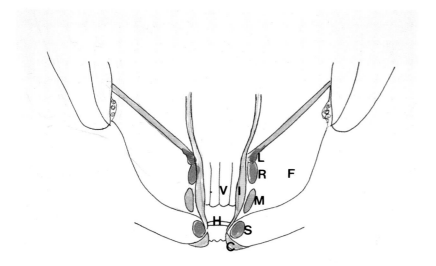

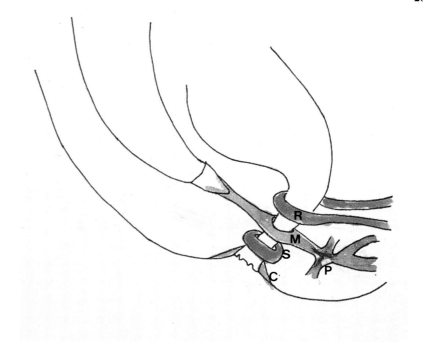

**200** The arrangements of the anal sphincters. An intrinsic involuntary smooth muscle sphincter consisting of a condensation of circular muscle fibres (I) extends down to the white line of Hilton (H). External to the wall of the ano-rectal canal are (from superficial to deep) the corrugator cutis ani (C), the subcutaneous ring-like portion of the external sphincter (S), and then in the ischiorectal fossa (F) the superficial external anal sphincter (M), which is also attached to the coccyx and the perineal body (P). Deep to this is the deep external anal sphincter which forms a sling at the ano-rectal junction (R). This fuses above with the pubo-rectalis portion of the levator ani muscle (L), which is the main part of the pelvic diaphragm. The mucosal anal columns joining to each other below, as the anal valves, are indicated (V).

---

\*The subcutaneous muscle layer called the panniculus carnosis is well developed in many mammals but in man it has disappeared from most parts of the body, exceptions being the corrugator cutis ani, the dartos muscle in the scrotum, the subareolar muscle of the nipple, the scalp, face and platisma muscle in the neck.

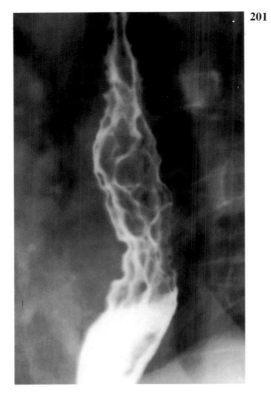

**201** Barium swallow showing the characteristic appearance of serpiginous filling defects due to oesophageal varices secondary to portal hypertension.

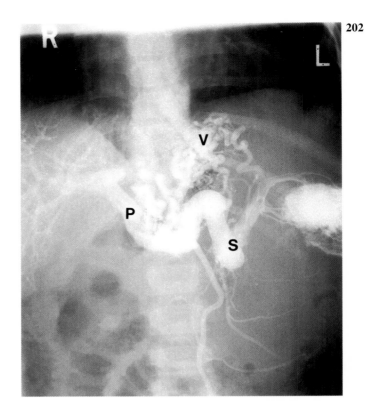

**202** A splenic venogram showing large varicose veins bending around the fundus of the stomach and into the oesophagus. Splenic vein (S), portal vein (P), varicosities (V).

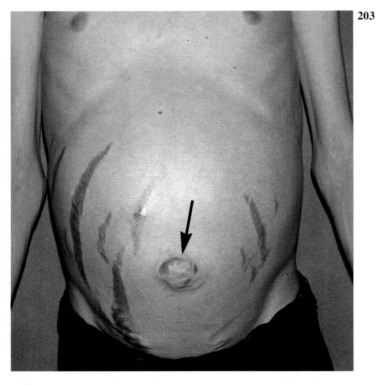

**203** A young patient with chronic active hepatitis with gross distension of the abdomen due to ascites. Note the striae of long-term corticosteroid treatment and huge collateral veins around the umbilicus called a "caput medusa" (arrow).

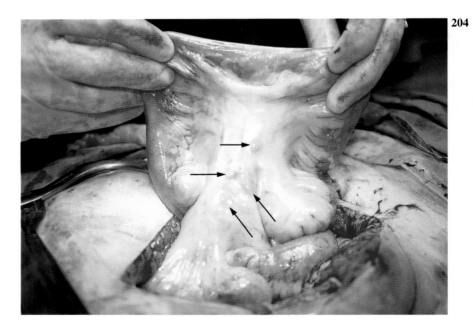

**204** A loop of ileum is lifted up. In the mesentery can be seen nodules produced by calcified mesenteric lymph nodes (arrows), the result of an old tuberculous infection.

At the upper and lower extremities of the portal venous watershed, posteriorly in the retroperitoneal space and anteriorly along the ligamentum teres, there are venous communications with the systemic veins which can become varicose in patients with portal hypertension.

**A** Oesophagus in the submucous layer – a source of lethal massive haemorrhage (**201, 202**).

**B** Ano-rectal haemorrhoids secondary to portal hypertension.

**C** The retroperitoneal space.

**D** Periumbilical – caput medusa (**203**).

The lymphatics draining the viscera first pass into the perivisceral nodes and then along the arteries to the preaortic nodes (**204, 205**). Thence to the *cisterna chyli* and *thoracic duct*, which passes behind the aorta and reaches the posterior surface of the oesophagus, crossing from right to left to reach the *left subclavian vein*. Malignant cells can pass retrograde at this point into a *supraclavicular lymph node*, the Node of Virchow\* and Sign of Troisier† (**206, 207**).

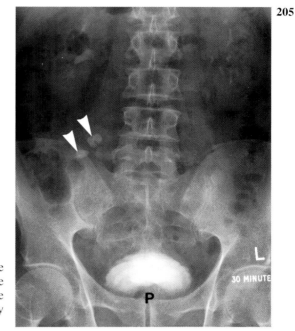

**205**  A straight X-ray of a patient who has had an intravenous urogram. The prostate (P) is enlarged and is indenting the bladder which has trabeculation. The renal calyceal systems can be seen. In addition there are two large opacities in the right iliac fossa which are calcified old tuberculous lymph nodes in the mesentery (arrows).

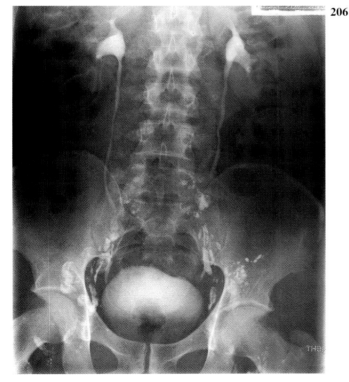

**206**  A lymphogram performed by cannulating lymphatics in the feet. Markedly enlarged lymph nodes can be seen alongside the aorta. In addition intravenous contrast has filled both renal collecting systems; (the ureters are displaced laterally by the abnormal para-aortic nodes).

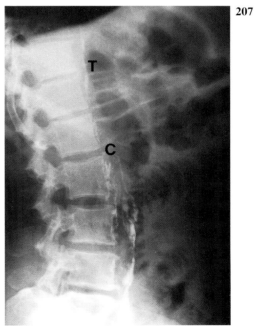

**207**  A lateral view of a normal lymphogram showing nodes in front of and behind the aorta. Note the normal cisterna chyli (C) and thoracic duct (T) more cranially.

\*Virchow, Rudolf Ludwig Karl (1821-1902) Professor of Pathological Anatomy – Berlin.
†Troisier Charles Émile (1844-1919) Professor of Pathology – Paris.

# The Spleen

The spleen lies in the left hypochondrium. It is a fragile vascular organ which destroys old red and white blood cells and platelets. It contains much lymphoid tissue and is therefore an important component of the immune system. The organ is convex shaped on the diaphragmatic surface where it is related to the left 9th, 10th, and 11th ribs posteriorly (**208, 209**). Removal of the spleen causes the platelets and neutrophil count to rise and leaves the individual susceptible to infection. This is a special danger in children, who have a tendency to succumb to pneumococcal septicaemia after splenectomy.

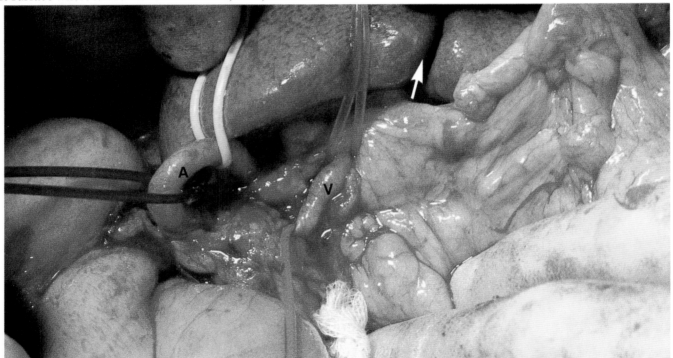

**208**  A photograph of a splenic hilum showing tortuous splenic artery (A) with a blue and white sling and a splenic vein (V) with two translucent slings below. The notch in the spleen (arrow) can easily be seen.

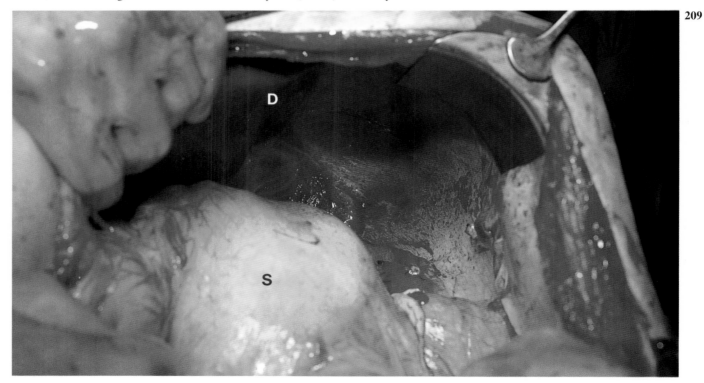

**209**  The left dome of the diaphragm (D) above and the greater curve of the stomach below (S). This is the splenic fossa after the spleen has been removed.

# The Pancreas

The pancreas is shaped like a tadpole with a large head and thick tail (**210**). The head lies in the concavity of the C of the duodenum to the right of the midline. There is a cleft at the neck where the uncinate horn-shaped process curls around the superior mesenteric vessels (**211**). The body of the pancreas crosses the aorta obliquely and passes upwards and to the left to become the tail which lies in front of the upper part of the left renal hilum, where it ends close to the hilum of the spleen. The greater curve of the stomach and the hilum of the spleen, the upper pole of the left kidney, the splenic flexure of the colon and the tail of the pancreas are all close together. Their relationship is maintained by folds of peritoneum, in particular, the gastrosplenic omentum, lienorenal ligament and peritoneum overlying the tail of the pancreas, the splenic hilum and the splenic flexure

of the colon. The pancreas arises from the foregut as two buds, each with their own duct, which fuse and usually communicate. The final duct arrangement varies but usually is as follows. The whole organ is drained by the main duct via the duct of Wirsung* into the ampulla of Vater (**212**). In 10% of cases, the foetal arrangement persists, the body and tail of the pancreas drain via the accessory pancreatic duct of Santorini† opening into the duodenum 2 cm proximal to the sphincter of Oddi, and the uncinate process drains by the duct of Wirsung into the ampulla of Vater. This is called *pancreas divisum* (**213**). The splenic artery supplies the body and tail of the pancreas. The superior pancreatico-duodenal branch of the gastroduodenal artery and the inferior pancreatico-duodenal branches of the superior mesenteric artery supply the head and uncinate process (**214**).

**210**

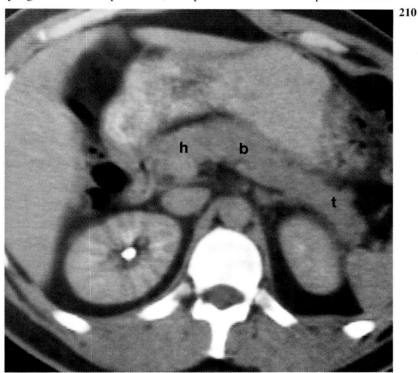

**210** A CT scan of the abdomen showing the head (h), body (b) and tail (t) of the pancreas. Also clearly seen are the two kidneys and the right lobe of the liver and the stomach.

**212**

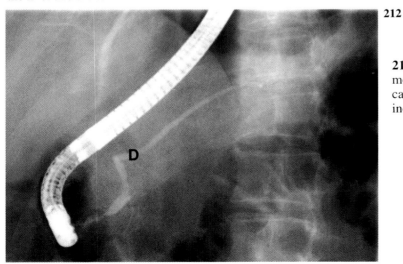

**211**

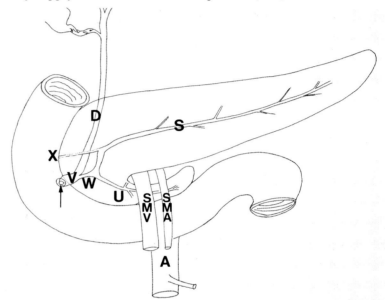

**211** A diagram of the usual arrangement of the pancreatic ducts. The body and tail of the pancreas drain through the main duct, which is the remnant of the duct of Santorini (S), which has joined the duct of Wirsung (W) from the uncinate process in the head (U). This opens into the ampulla of Vater (V) into which the common bile duct (D) also usually opens. The exit into the duodenum is guarded by the sphincter of Oddi (arrow). The ampulla of Vater can be seen from the duodenal surface. The position of the residual duct of Santorini which persists in some 10% of cases is indicated (X). The superior mesenteric vessels (SMV and SMA) and aorta (A) are shown.

**212** Endoscopic pancreatogram. The endoscope has been passed through the mouth to the duodenum and the ampulla of Vater and pancreatic ducts have been cannulated. The angulation of the pancreatic duct (D) is clearly shown, as indicated in the previous diagram.

*Wirsung, Johann Georg (1600-1643) Professor of Anatomy – Padua.
†Santorini, Giovanni Domenico (1681-1737) Professor of Anatomy and Medicine – Venice.

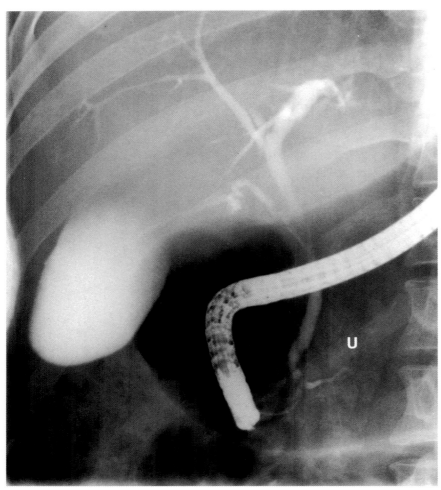

**213** Endoscopic pancreatogram only filling the uncinate process (U) and the biliary system. The rest of the pancreas will drain through the accessory pancreatic duct. This is a case of pancreas divisum (same case as **191**).

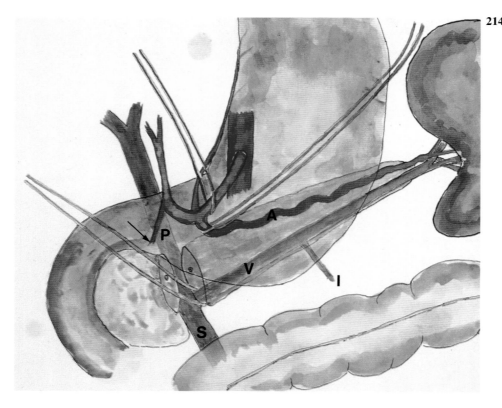

**214** A diagram to show the relation of the pancreas to the stomach, duodenum, portal vein and hilum of the spleen. The blood supply to the tail and body of the pancreas comes from the splenic artery (A). The head of the pancreas receives its blood supply from the gastro-duodenal (arrow) via the superior pancreaticoduodenal branch and the superior mesenteric via the inferior pancreatico-duodenal branch. The point of section shown in the diagram is the junction of the two blood supplies of the pancreas and it happens to overlie the formation of the portal vein (P). It is important surgically because in partial resection of the pancreas the division usually occurs in this plane. Splenic vein (V), inferior mesenteric vein (I), superior mesenteric vein (S).

# The Liver and Gall Bladder

The liver is an irregularly shaped organ resembling a pear on its side cut obliquely in the longitudinal plane (**215**). The right and left lobes are fused together at a plane that passes from the gall bladder fossa to the vena cava. The falciform ligament, its fissure and the fissure for the ligamentum venosum make the important surgical division between the medial and lateral segments of the left lobe (**216**). The quadrate lobe lies between the gall bladder and the falciform ligament. The caudate lobe lies mainly in the medial segment of the left lobe posteriorly (**217**). It has a tail-like caudate process which lies behind the portal vein at the upper border of the aditus of the lesser sac. These lobes are surface landmarks of the liver, but the remaining lobar subdivisions of the liver are not important surgically because their vascular arrangements do not readily permit dissection. The superior diaphragmatic surface is convex. The anterior edge of the liver passes on the right side parallel to the right costal margin and under the left costal margin to the wedge shaped extremity of the left lobe.

The gall bladder, a muscular, pear-shaped organ, lies in a fossa in the under surface of the right lobe. Its fundus is anterior and to the right. The narrow body extends towards the hilum of the liver to a widened *pouch of Hartmann*\* leading to the *cystic duct* which joins the common hepatic duct to form the common bile duct. Within the cystic duct is a spiral fold of mucosa which acts as a valve, the *valve of Heister*†, permitting passive flow of bile into the gall bladder by

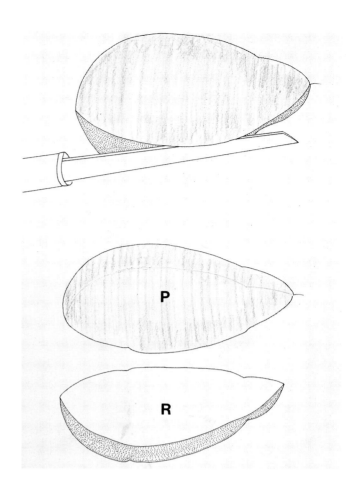

**215** Diagram of the approximate shape of the liver (P), being that of a pear that has been sliced to have the lower portion removed, as shown (R).

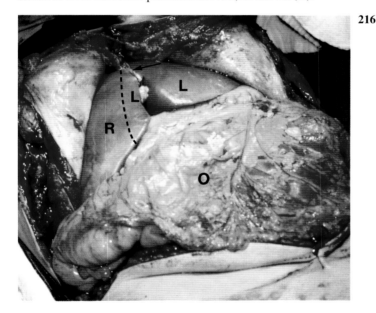

**216** The liver displayed. A bilateral subcostal incision has been made with extension vertically up to the xiphisternum. The falciform ligament (arrow) has been divided. The right (R) and left (L) lobes of the liver can be seen together with the omentum (O). The dotted line marks the boundary between the right and left lobes.

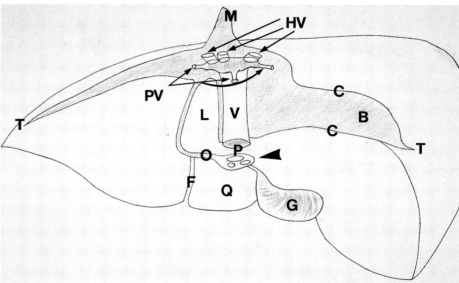

**217** Diagram of the liver viewed from behind, showing the vena cava (V) and gall bladder (G). Between the gall bladder and the fissure of the ligamentum teres (F) is the quadrate lobe (Q). The lesser omentum (O) is shown passing into the fissure for the ligamentum venosum with the structures in its free edge (arrowhead), the portal vein posteriorly, hepatic artery to the left, and common bile duct to the right. The peritoneal reflections are indicated with the shaded area between them; the right and left triangular ligaments (T), the falciform (M) and coronary ligaments (C) and the bare area (B). Between the vena cava and lesser omentum is the caudate process (P) leading to the caudate lobe (L). The three hepatic veins and three phrenic veins are shown arrowed (HV) and (PV).

\*Hartmann, Henri Albert Charles Antoine (1860-1952) Professor of Surgery – Paris.
†Heister, Lorenz (1683-1758) Professor of Anatomy and Surgery – Helmstädt.

hydrostatic pressure when the sphincter of Oddi is closed. Thus the gall bladder fills with bile, which is concentrated tenfold, by absorption of water. When fatty food enters the duodenum, the enteric hormone, cholecystokinin, is released into the portal venous system from the duodenal mucosa. This together with vagal activity, causes the gall bladder to contract which automatically opens the spiral valve.

Some of the gall bladder veins and small arteries pass directly into and from the liver through the gall bladder bed. Others pass alongside the cystic duct to the portal vein in the hilum of the liver. The main cystic artery is usually a branch of the right hepatic passing to Hartmann's pouch behind and above the cystic duct. The area between the cystic artery, cystic duct and common hepatic duct (Calot's* triangle) is important in surgical practice because the main bile duct can be damaged if the anatomy is not clearly defined.

Most of the liver is covered with visceral peritoneum fused to the thin fibrous envelope of the liver, (*Glisson's† capsule*). The obliterated left umbilical vein passes as the ligamentum teres to the liver in the midline, the anatomical junction of medial and lateral segments of the left lobe. It is surrounded by peritoneum forming the free edge of the sickle-shaped falciform ligament which continues over the convex diaphragmatic surface of the left lobe. The leaves of peritoneum diverge on the upper surface of the liver. The right leaf forms the *coronary ligament* and the left leaf, the left triangular ligament. This connects the left lobe of the liver to the diaphragm and if it is divided, the left lobe can be lifted up and forwards to reveal the lesser omentum passing between the lesser curve of the stomach and the back of the left lobe of the liver, where it is attached to the fissure for the ligamentum venosum, in the midline (**48**, page 26). It contains hepatic branches of anterior and posterior vagus nerves from the region of the oesophago-gastric junction.

The vagi also give off two long, fine, longitudinal running anterior and posterior nerves of Latarget (**153**, page 62), which also lie in the lesser omentum. The branches from these passing to the body of the stomach are cut in a highly selective vagotomy. The nerves of Latarget end in the pyloric antrum, where they control the motor function that opens the pylorus. The vagi continue posteriorly to give branches to the coeliac plexus, from which they are conveyed together with sympathetic fibres along the visceral and segmental arteries to supply structures derived from the foregut and midgut as far distally as the splenic flexure of the colon. Branches are also distributed to the adrenals and kidneys.

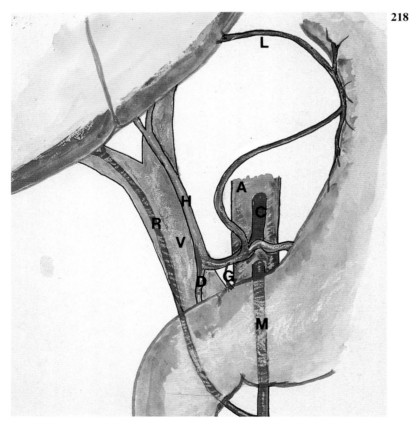

**218** Common vascular anomalies in the blood supply to the liver. The major left hepatic branch is shown coming off the left gastric artery (L) which occurs in 23% of cases, and a major right hepatic artery is shown coming off the superior mesenteric (R), which has a 17% incidence. This vessel usually passes behind the portal vein (V) but can be in front of that structure. Arteries indicated: aorta (A), coeliac (C), right gastric (G), gastro-duodenal (D), hepatic (H) and superior mesenteric (M).

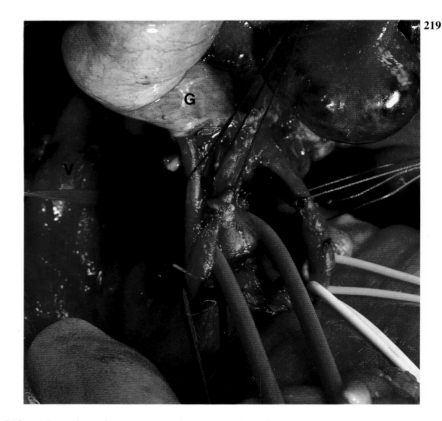

**219** Dissection of the structures in the free edge of the lesser omentum. The gall bladder (G) and vena cava (V). A blue sling is passed around the common bile duct, a red sling around the portal vein, a yellow sling around the hepatic artery, and a white sling around the gastro-duodenal artery.

*Calot, Jean Francis (1861-1944) Surgeon – France.
†Glisson, Francis (1597-1677) Regius Professor of Physics – Cambridge.

The lesser omentum may contain an aberrant left hepatic artery, a branch of the left gastric (in 23% of cases) (**218**). The lesser omentum forms part of the anterior wall of the lesser sac – as it is traced inferiorly and to the right it ends as the free edge containing the hepatic artery, the bile duct and portal vein (**219, 220**). There are also numerous lymphatics, a few lymph nodes and nerve fibres from the coeliac plexus. In 17% of cases the main arterial blood supply to the right lobe of the liver is a branch of the superior mesenteric, which passes posterior to the portal vein (**221-223**).

Continuing the course of the coronary ligament to the right of the midline, it passes from the liver to the diaphragm and to the right where it turns back on itself as the right triangular ligament. It then runs posteriorly away from the anterior leaf to behind the vena cava near the diaphragm leaving a triangular portion of the posterior diaphragmatic surface of the liver in direct contact with the diaphragm. This is called the *bare area* of the liver, since it is not covered by peritoneum (**224**). Some lymphatics and blood vessels pass directly from the bare area of liver surface to the diaphragm and into the chest, anastomosing with those in the pleura.

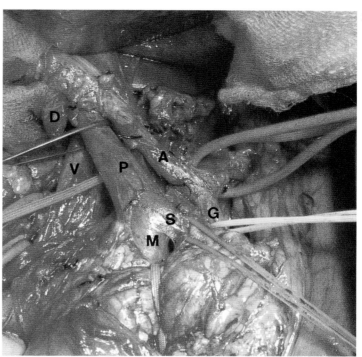

**220**   High power of a dissection of the structures in the free edge of the lesser omentum. Portal vein (P), splenic vein (S), superior mesenteric vein (M), gastro-duodenal (G), hepatic artery (A), upper end of common bile duct (D) cut and vena cava (V).

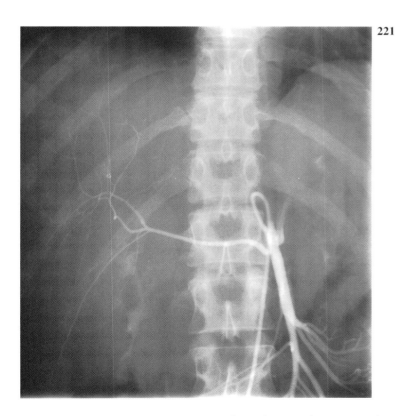

**221**   The right hepatic artery arising from the superior mesenteric artery in a case of liver tumour.

**222**   Same patient as **221**; the tumour in the left lobe of the liver is stretching the left hepatic arterial branches (cannula in coeliac artery).

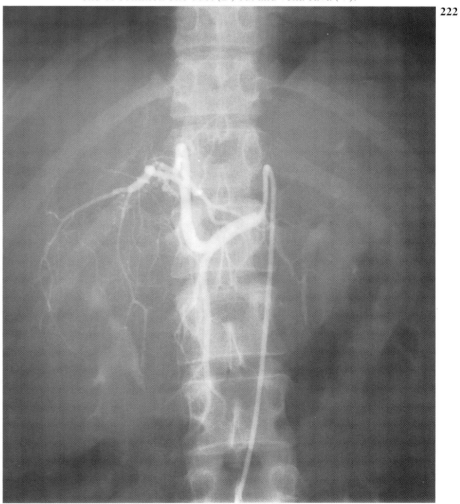

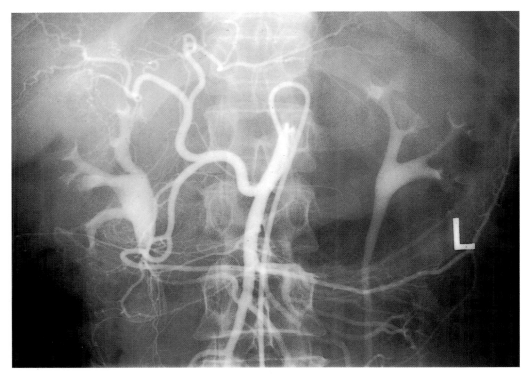

**223**   The main hepatic artery arising from the superior mesenteric artery.

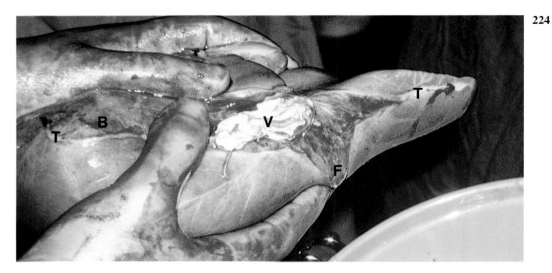

**224**   The cooled but live liver removed from chilled saline for transplantation. It is orientated so that the convex diaphragmatic surface lies under the surgeon's right hand. His index finger is pointing to the falciform ligament (F). The right and left triangular ligaments (T) can be seen. The surgeon's right thumb lies on the bare area of the liver (B). The vena cava and a cuff of diaphragm lie between the surgeon's right thumb and index finger (V).

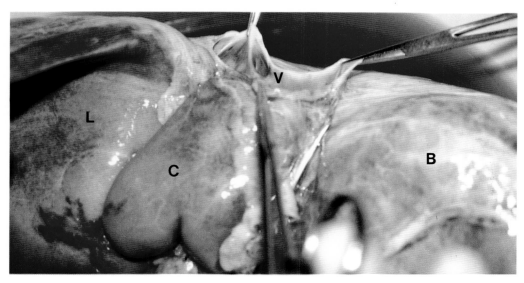

**225**   The hepatic veins entering the vena cava (V) just before the vena cava passes through the diaphragm. Left lobe (L), caudate lobe (C), bare area (B).

The inferior vena cava after receiving the two renal veins reaches the under surface of the liver. It lies in a sagittal cleft between the right and left lobes where it receives the *right adrenal vein*, a variable number of lumbar veins and some accessory hepatic veins, including a vein draining the caudate lobe. The vena cava ends its intra-abdominal course at the diaphragm where it receives the main right and left hepatic veins (**225**).

The liver consists microscopically of lobules, each surrounded by a thin layer of fibrous tissue. Between the lobules are the portal triads conveying the radicals of the main vessels from the free edge of the lesser omentum, namely the hepatic artery, portal vein and bile duct (**226-229**). There are some connections between the hepatic artery and portal vein, but the main flow of blood in both of these vessels is through the vascular sinusoids of the lobule to the central vein, a tributary of the hepatic vein. Bile is secreted by hepatocytes into the biliary canaliculae, which, like the tributaries of a river, join to form the main bile ducts.

The gross vascular intrahepatic anatomy is important because of surgical considerations in hepatic resections. In the free edge of the lesser omentum the common hepatic artery and portal vein bifurcate. The junction of the right and left main hepatic ducts is a little closer to the hilum. These three structures then pass to the right and left lobes fanning out from the hilum and dividing into major and minor branches. The hepatic venous tributaries pass upwards and posteriorly. There are three main hepatic veins, the right, left and the median sagittal vein which usually joins the left, (60%) but may enter the

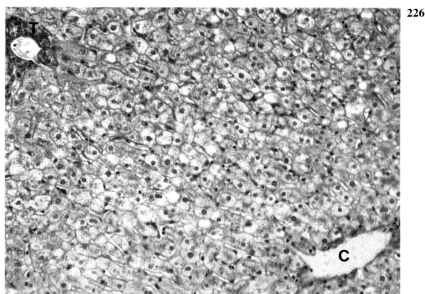

**226**

**226** Histology of the liver showing a portal triad of the bile duct, hepatic artery and portal vein radicles in the top left hand corner (T) and the central vein in the bottom right hand corner (C). The columns of liver cells between these structures form the lobule.

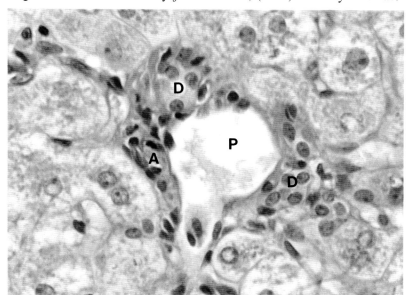

**227**

**227** The high power view of the portal triad, showing radicles of portal vein (P), hepatic artery (A) and bile ducts (D).

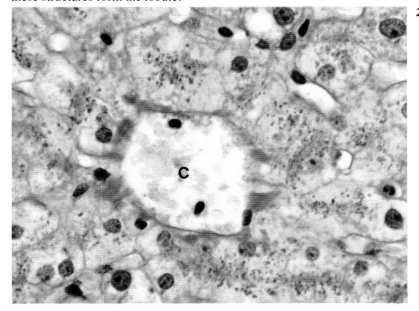

**228**

**228** High power view of the central vein (C).

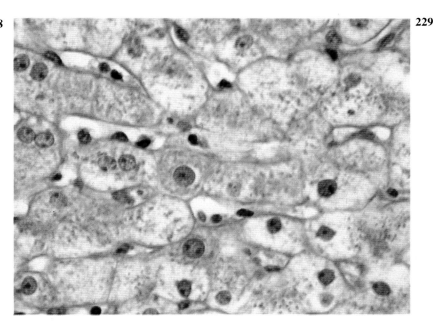

**229**

**229** High power view of the columns of liver cells with the vascular sinusoids between them. Some of the cells lining these sinusoids are modified macrophages called Kupffer cells.

inferior vena cava independently (**230**). The hepatic veins have very short extra-hepatic courses before reaching the cava at an angle of 45° (**231**). They are vulnerable to trauma if the liver receives a blunt injury and is dislocated away from the diaphragm. Three phrenic veins *right*, *left* and *posterior* draining the diaphragm, enter the cava at the same level as the hepatic veins (**232**). The hepatic veins within the liver run at right angles to the direction of the structures of the portal triad. These two courses have been likened to the crossing of the fingers of two hands (by Fagarasanu*) (**233**). Thus, when the liver substance is cut the blood vessels and bile ducts are often divided tangentially, in which case control is best achieved by sutures rather than simple ligatures which tend to cut out. Although local suture and

**230**

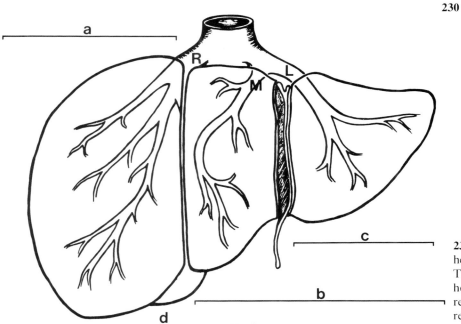

**230**   Diagram of the main venous drainage of the liver. There is a main right hepatic vein (R), a median sagittal vein (M), and a main left hepatic vein (L). The main types of hepatic resection based on the venous drainage are: right hepatic lobectomy (a); left hepatic lobectomy (b); left lateral segment resection (c) and right hepatic lobectomy together with left medial segment resection-trisegmentectomy (d).

**231**

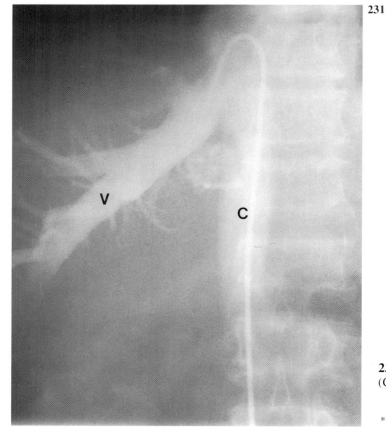

**231**   Venogram of the right hepatic vein system (V) draining into the inferior vena cava (C). The angle of junction of the hepatic vein to the vena cava is approximately 45°.

*Fagarasanu, I. Contemporary Rumanian Surgeon.

wedge resections of the liver are possible, the standard operations for severe trauma and cancer are right lobectomy, left lobectomy, left lateral segment removal and right lobectomy, together with left medial segment removal. Consideration of the vascular anatomy explains the rationale of these procedures (234–242). Other major segmental resections are seldom possible without damaging the central vital vessels.

The lymphatic drainage of the liver is mainly to hilar nodes, then to the pre-aortic nodes and on to the thoracic duct (243).

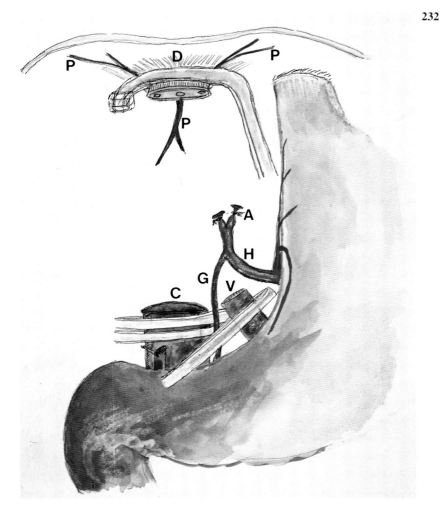

**232**   Diagram of the hepatic fossa with the liver removed as for a transplant. There is a clamp on the vena cava including a portion of diaphragm (D). The right, left and posterior phrenic veins can be seen draining into the vena cava at this point (P). Below two clamps are applied to the vena cava (C), one clamp to the portal vein (V). The right and left main hepatic arteries are ligated and divided (A). The common hepatic (H) with its right and left branches tied and gastro-duodenal (G) arteries are shown. The common bile duct, coloured green, has been cut across and there is a small suture marking its position.

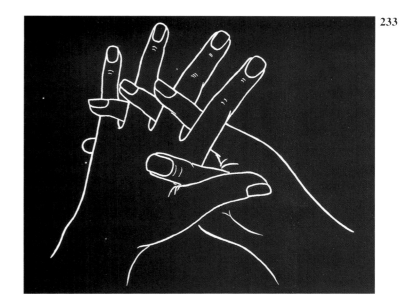

**233**   The relationship of inflow structures of portal vein, hepatic artery and bile duct tributaries to the venous drainage shown by the crossing of fingers to be approximately at right angles to each other. This is important surgically since the vessels tend to be cut tangentially and need to be suture-ligated so that the blood vessels and bile ducts are securely controlled.

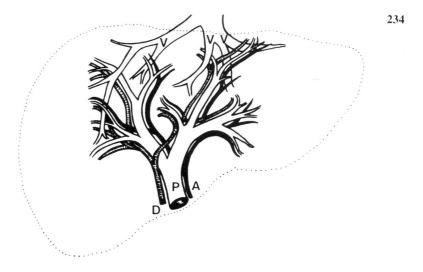

**234**   Diagram of the distribution of the inflow structures of hepatic artery (A), portal vein (P) and bile duct drainage (D) in relation to the venous outflow (V).

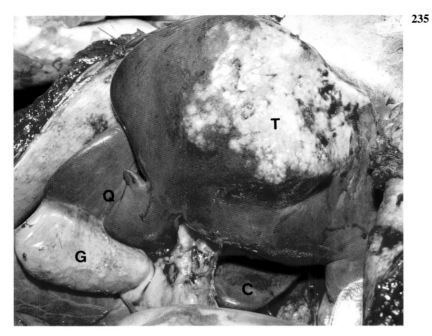

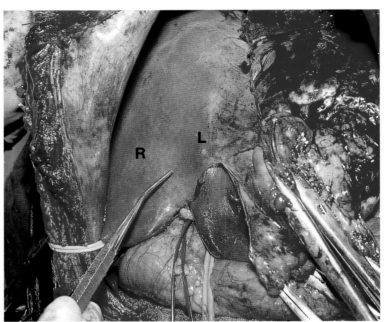

**235**   Tumour of the left lobe of the liver (T). The liver has been dissected and the under-surface lifted up. The tumour, coloured white, is easily seen. The gall bladder is on the left (G). Between the gall bladder and the tumour is the quadrate lobe (Q) and behind the lesser omentum is the caudate lobe (C).

**236**   The left lobe of the liver has been separated from the surrounding structures by division of its peritoneal attachments, which are clamped. The probe indicates the boundary between the pink right lobe (R) and the purple devascularized left lobe (L).

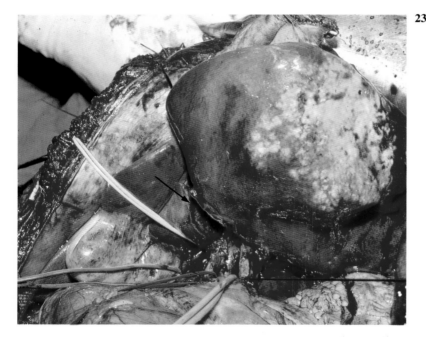

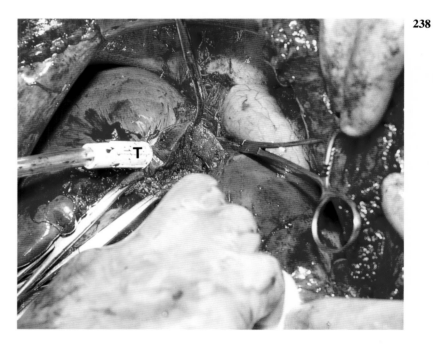

**237**   The left branch of the hepatic artery and the left branch of the portal vein have been ligated, allowing relatively bloodless dissection between the lateral segment of the left lobe and the rest of the liver (arrow).

**238**   A tourniquet (T) has been passed around the remaining liver tissue at the junction of the lateral and medical segments of the left lobe.

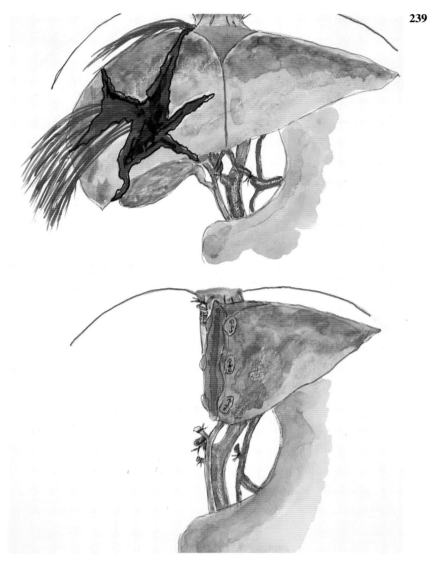

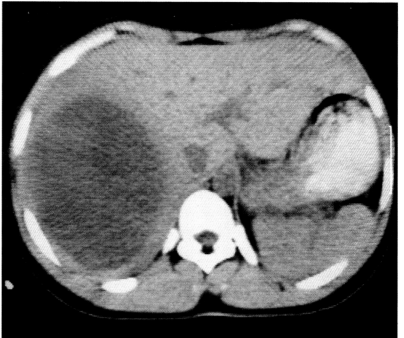

**240** CT scan of a patient with a tumour in the right lobe of the liver, at least 12 cm in diameter.

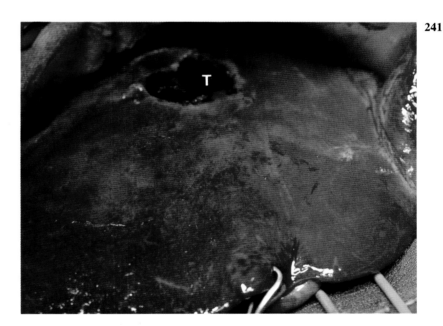

**239** Diagram of hepatic trauma which commonly results from a road traffic accident with the steering wheel crushing the right lobe of the liver and causing it to fracture in a stellate manner. If haemorrhage cannot be prevented by simple means, it may be necessary to remove the right lobe of the liver as shown in the lower diagram, with the right branches of the hepatic artery, portal vein and hepatic duct ligated and divided together with the main right hepatic vein. Sutures are indicated passing through the remaining stump of the liver through buttons made of fibrin to prevent them cutting through liver tissue.

**241** The right lobe of the liver has been mobilized. The tumour (T) is ulcerating the surface of the liver and is covered with blood clot.

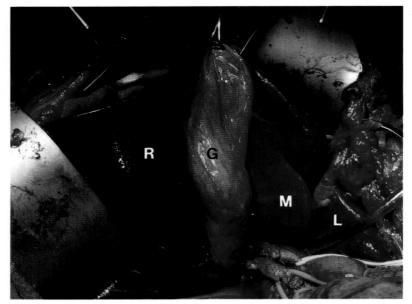

**242** The right main hepatic artery has been ligated and the right lobe of the liver has now turned a dusky colour (R). It will be removed together with the gall bladder (G) through the plane of the gall bladder bed. Left lobe medial segment (M), lateral segment (L).

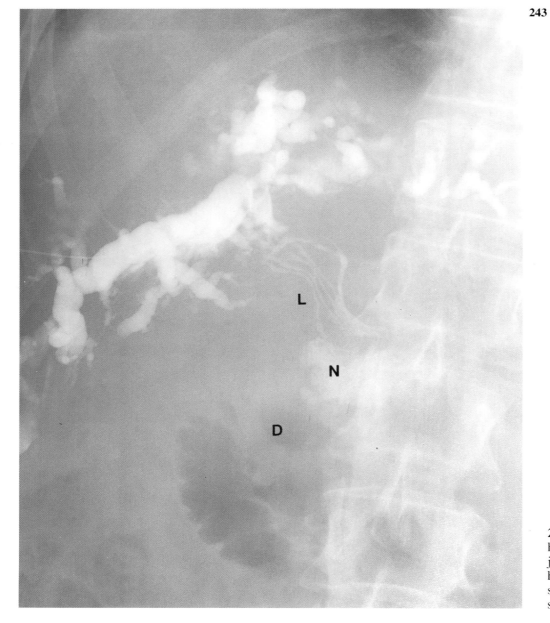

**243** Percutaneous cholangiogram showing dilated intra-hepatic bile ducts due to an obstructing tumour at the junction of the main right and left hepatic ducts. Contrast has passed into the periportal lymphatic vessels (L) along-side the portal vein en route to lymph nodes (N) lying superior to the first part of the duodenum (D).

# 4 The Organs Supplied by the Lateral Aortic Branches and the Pelvic Vessels

The topography of the abdominal viscera, the aorta and inferior vena cava and their segmental branches will now be considered.

The aorta and vena cava lie side by side in their course from the diaphragm to the front of the body of L4 where the aorta divides and gives off a small *median sacral* branch, which passes down in front of the sacrum to the rectum; the vena cava commences in front of the body of L5 by the junction of two common iliac veins (**244**). The aorta, 2-2.5 cm in diameter, has a powerful pulsation; the cava, soft, bluish in colour and collapsible is slightly flattened anteriorly and posteriorly so that in cross section it is ellipsoid measuring some 2.5 cm by 1.5 cm.

At the upper border of L1 the aorta passes under the crura of the diaphragm and the median arcuate ligament. It lies in front of and to the left of the lumbar vertebral bodies giving off two phrenic arteries at the origin of the coeliac trunk (**245**). These vessels also contribute to the supply of the adrenal glands (see page 99). Segmental lumbar vessels arise and pass around the bodies of each of the lumbar vertebrae to help supply the terminal spinal cord at L1 and the *cauda equina* below. The two renal vessels leave the aorta at L1, the same level as the superior mesenteric origin, and pass laterally to the renal hila, giving off adrenal branches (**246, 247**). The adrenals also receive small arteries direct from the aorta, so these little glands usually have three distinct arteries, from the phrenic, renal and aorta. Below the renal arteries are the origins of the gonadal vessels which pass laterally down and forwards to supply the ovaries in the female and the testicles in the male.

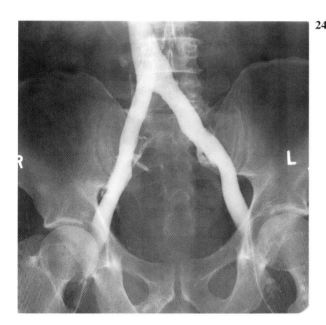

**244** Venogram showing both common iliac veins joining to form the vena cava over the body of L 5.

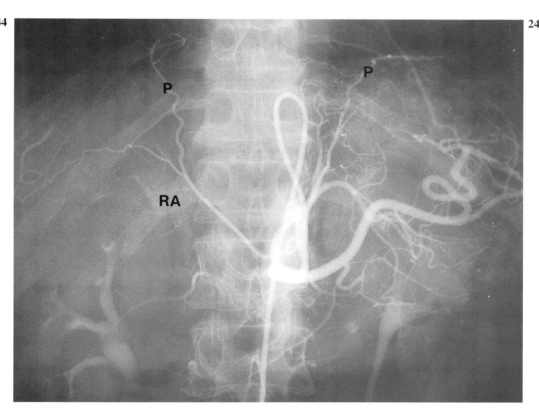

**245** Selective splenic arteriogram showing both inferior phrenic arteries (P) and a branch outlining the right adrenal gland (RA).

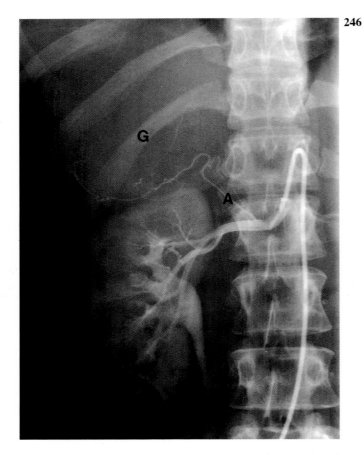

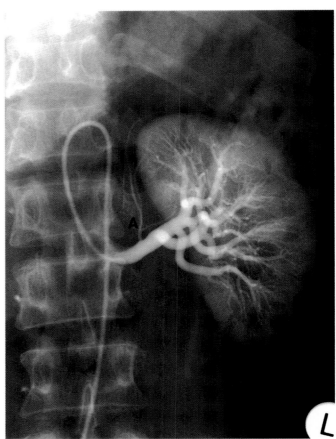

**246** Angiogram of the right renal artery showing an adrenal artery (A) supplying an enlarged right adrenal gland (G).

**247** Angiogram of the left renal artery showing an adrenal artery (A) supplying a normal adrenal gland.

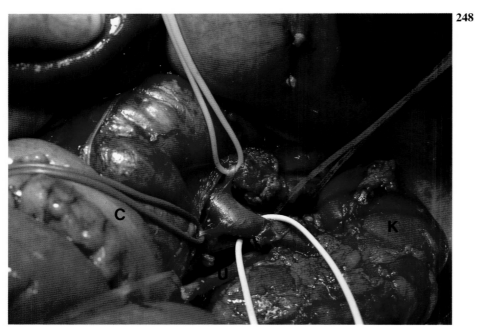

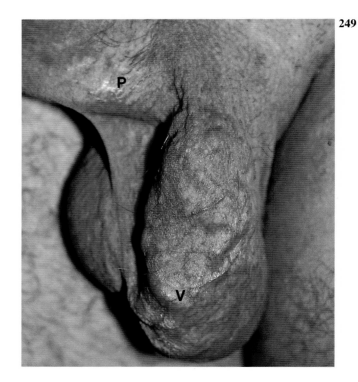

**248** Dissection of the left kidney (K) viewed from the left hand side. Slings: white, renal vein; brown, gonadal; yellow, adrenal; colon (C); ureter (U).

**249** Varicocoele of the left scrotum (V), root of penis (P). A left varicocoele is rarely secondary to the tumour blocking the left gonadal vein.

The vena cava is formed at the junction of the two common iliac veins behind and below the aortic bifurcation to the right of and in front of the body of L5. It ascends with the aortic wall closely applied to its left side, receiving segmental lumbar veins. The right gonadal vein enters the front of the vena cava; on the left the gonadal vein enters the renal vein (**248**). Tumour in the left renal vein from a renal cell cancer can block the left gonadal vein. Very rarely this causes a left *varicocoele* (varicose veins in the pampiniform plexus in the scrotum), which when the patient stands looks and feels like a bag of worms (**249**). Usually there is no sinister cause of a varicocoele. The left renal vein also receives the *left adrenal vein* and a lumbar vein. It then passes in front of the aorta, below the duodenum, to reach the cava (**250**). The left renal vein, 5 cm long, is an important relation to the neck of an abdominal aneurysm (**459**). The right renal vein is only 2 cm long (**251**). It usually has no tributaries, the *right adrenal vein* passing directly into the cava. The vena cava continues cephalward to reach the inferior surface of the liver. It passes through the liver, receiving the hepatic and phrenic veins before passing through the diaphragm at the level of T9 to enter the pericardium within the chest, where it joins the right atrium (**252**).

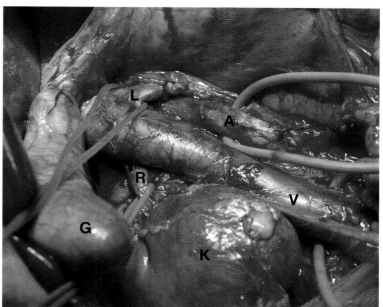

250

**250** An extensive Kocher's manoeuvre. The vena cava (V) can be seen running obliquely across the picture. Above it is the aorta (A) and the left renal vein (L) can be seen crossing the aorta. It is controlled with a blue sling. The gall bladder (G) and the liver are on the left of the picture. Right kidney (K), right renal vein (R).

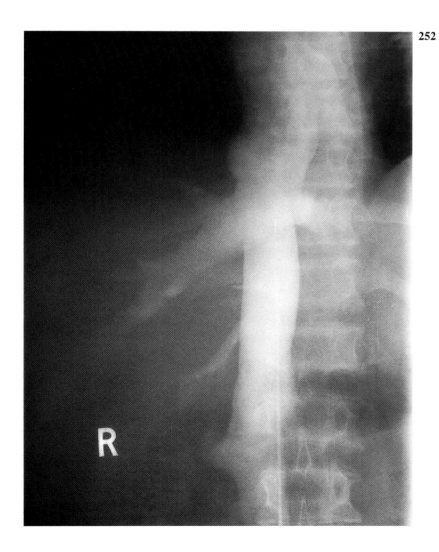

252

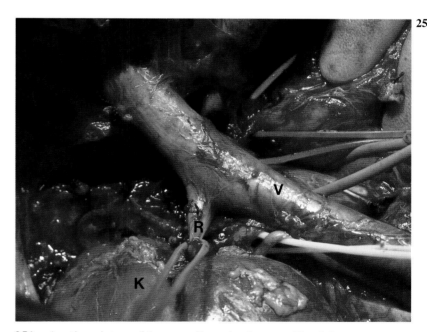

251

**251** Another picture of the same dissection later on. The right renal vein (R) is controlled with a brown sling which can be clearly seen. Vena cava (V), right kidney (K).

**252** Venogram showing the vena cava passing up within the liver and the diaphragm. The hepatic veins join just below the diaphragm and there is a separate vein from the caudate lobe inferiorly. The right atrium is opacified above the diaphragm.

The common iliac arteries, 4 cm in length, pass in front of the corresponding veins. They give off no branches except for their terminal bifurcation into internal and external iliacs (253, 254). The iliac veins accompany the arteries. The ureters cross in front of the common iliac arterial bifurcations, passing from above laterally to below medially. The external iliac arteries run along the pelvic brim, passing to the lateral side of the corresponding veins. Just before going under the inguinal ligament to become the femoral artery each external iliac gives off its only branch, the inferior epigastric, which passes medially forwards and upwards around the medial margin of the internal inguinal ring so that herniae arising lateral to it are indirect, while those arising medial to it are direct. This vessel cannot be felt on clinical examination. It passes behind the rectus muscle and in front of the arcuate line of the inferior margin of the posterior rectus sheath. It supplies the rectus muscle and anastomoses with the superior epigastric artery, a terminal branch of the internal mammary artery (internal thoracic), after the latter branch has given off the musculo-phrenic artery, which supplies the anterior portion of the diaphragm.

The internal iliac or hypogastric arteries pass medially inferiorly and posteriorly into the pelvis dividing after 2 cm into anterior and posterior divisions. From the anterior are given the vessels supplying the pelvic viscera; the posterior division leaves the pelvis and supplies the gluteal region. In the foetus the main continuation of the internal iliac artery is the umbilical artery, which becomes obliterated as the fibrous cord of the medial umbilical ligament. The proximal portion of this remains as the superior vesical artery. The veins follow the arteries. There is a rich plexus of veins around the prostate which anastomose with sacral veins and receive the dorsal vein of the penis. These drain into the internal iliac veins.

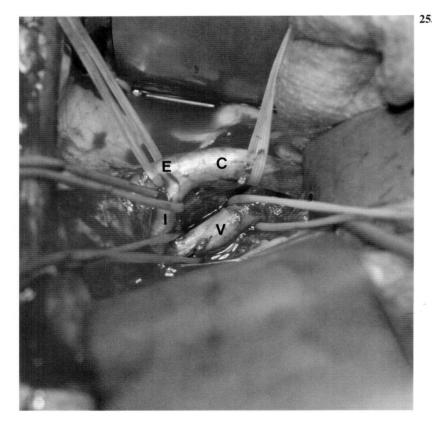

**253**

**253** The right iliac vessels viewed from the left. There is a blue sling around the external iliac vein passing inferior and medially towards the inguinal ligament. The common iliac artery (C) divides into external (E) and internal (I) branches. A segment of the common iliac vein (V) is controlled with slings.

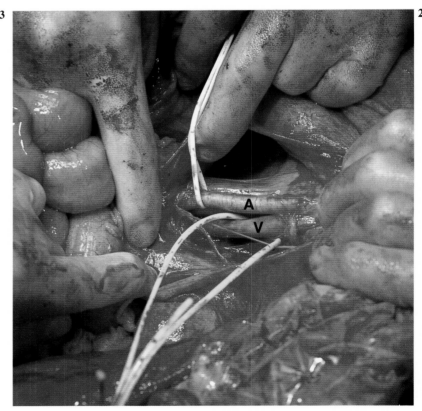

**254**

**254** The right common iliac vessels viewed from above. A yellow sling is around the vein (V) and a white sling is around the common iliac artery (A).

# The Paired Organs of the Abdomen and Pelvis

## The Adrenals

These are small wedge shaped glands 4 cm across lying antero-medial to the upper poles of the kidney. They have vital endocrine functions. They are strikingly yellow in colour, which aids their identification (**255**). They have an outer cortex responsible for the secretion of both mineralocorticoid and glucocorticoid hormones. The medulla secretes adrenaline and noradrenaline. The right adrenal is tucked behind the cava and has a short relatively wide lumened vein which drains into that vessel. The left adrenal lies above the left renal vein to which it is attached by a short draining vessel. The arterial supply comes from the renal and phrenic arteries and direct from the aorta (**256-258**).

**256-258** Three contiguous expanded CT images through the adrenal glands.

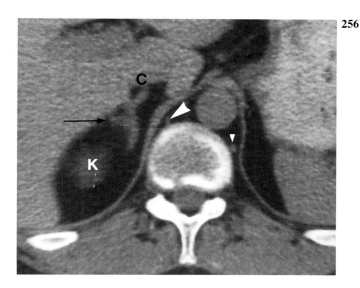

256

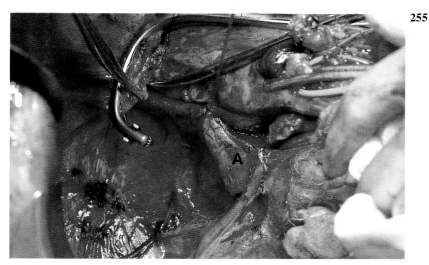

255

**255** Photograph of the hepatic fossa with the liver removed. There is a large curved clamp around the diaphragm enclosing the vena cava. In the middle of the field the yellow pyramidal shaped right adrenal gland can be seen (A). The adrenal vein has a ligature around it.

**256** The normal tri-limbed wedge shaped right adrenal gland (arrow) immediately behind the inferior vena cava (C) which is still closely abutting the caudate lobe of liver. See how it is antero-medial to the upper pole of the right kidney (K). Note azygos (large arrowhead) and hemi-azygos (small arrowhead) veins posteromedial to the right and left diaphragmatic crura respectively.

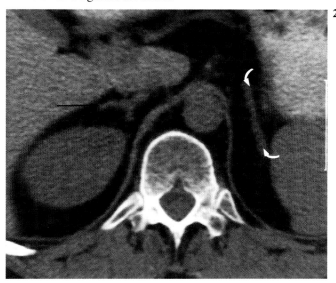

257

**257** The right adrenal is again clearly seen (straight arrow). The left adrenal is now seen as a long slit-shaped structure; the anterior and postero-medial limbs are confluent (between curved arrows).

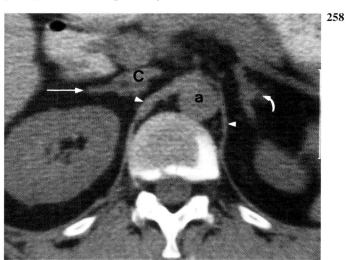

258

**258** The cava (C) is now separate from the caudate lobe. The most caudal portion of the right adrenal (straight arrow) is closely applied to the cava. The left adrenal (curved arrow) now assumes a tri-limbed shape. Note how the aorta (a) is still retrocrural at this stage. Arrowheads mark the crura.

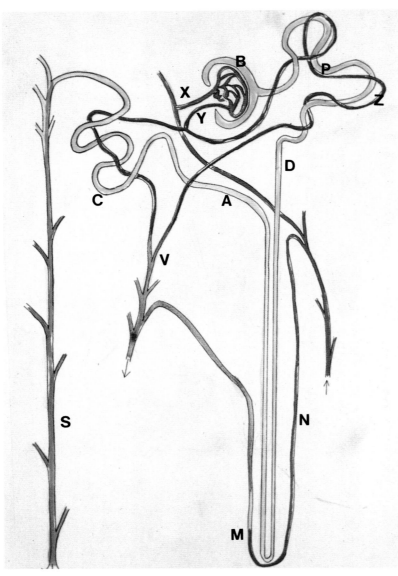

# The Kidneys

These are mirror images of each other, with a characteristic bean shape, but the left lies a little higher than the right. The lateral borders are convex and the medial concave; poles are both convex. The longitudinal measurement from pole to pole is 11-14 cm and across to the hilum 6 cm. Each kidney has approximately one million functioning units called nephrons. Each nephron has a glomerulus, which acts as a blood filter, supplied by an *afferent* and drained by an *efferent* arteriole. The efferent arterioles break up into peritubular capillaries (**259-261**). Both the glomeruli and the metabolically active tubules lie in the cortex of the kidney, which is darker in colour than the medulla when perfused with blood, but pale when the blood is washed out (**262-265**). The medulla contains the urinary collecting ducts, which open into the papillae (5 to 11 in number) at the tips of the pyramids. These project into the "champagne glass" shaped renal calyces which join the muscular pelvis, which is drained by the ureter. The pelvis and ureter are lined with transitional cell epithelium that resists the corrosive effects of urine.

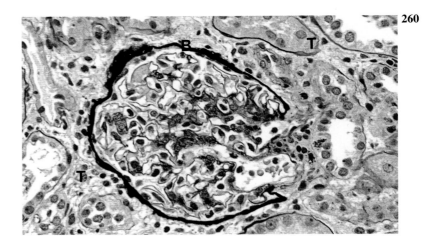

**260**  Histology of a glomerulus. Bowman's capsule (B) can be seen clearly. Renal tubules (T) surround the glomerulus.

**259**  Diagram of nephron. Filtrate from the blood flowing through the glomerulus passes through Bowman's* capsule (B), and thence into the proximal convoluted tubule (P). The route continues into the descending limb of the loop of Henle† (D) and back via the ascending limb (A) to the distal convoluted tubule (C); the collecting duct system (S) opens into the renal pyramid. The vascular pattern is shown first in red with an afferent artery (X) to the glomerulus itself and then the efferent artery (Y) which gives rise to peritubular capillaries (Z) which drain into the veins (V). There are also long descending (N) and ascending (M) arterioles and venules going from the cortex to the medulla and back.

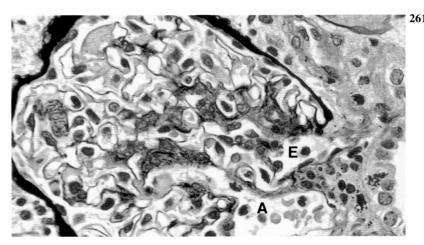

**261**  High power view of the glomerulus. Afferent arteriole (A), efferent arteriole (E).

---

*Bowman, Sir William Paget (1816-1902). Surgeon in Birmingham and London. Also Professor of Anatomy and Physiology, King's College Hospital, London.

†Henle, Freidrich Gustav Jakob (1809-1885). Professor of Anatomy, Zurich, Heidelberg and Göttingen.

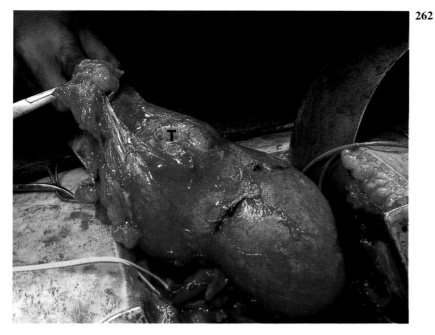

**262** The left kidney has been mobilized. There is a tumour (T) in the lower pole.

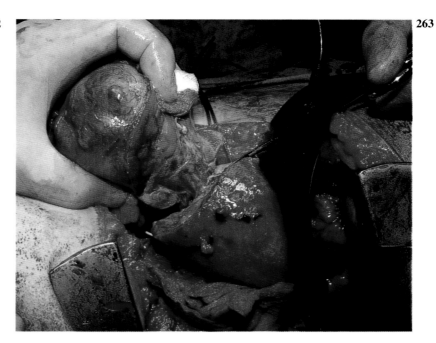

**263** The vessels have been temporarily clamped and the kidney incised so that the tumour can be removed.

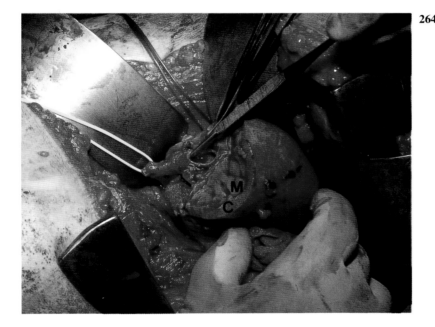

**264** The tumour has been removed. The cut parenchyma can be seen, the cortex (C) is red in colour, the medulla (M) leading to the pyramids is pale. There is a dark red junction between the cortex and the medulla outlining the pyramids. The probe is inside the renal pelvis with its tip inside the origin of the ureter (yellow sling).

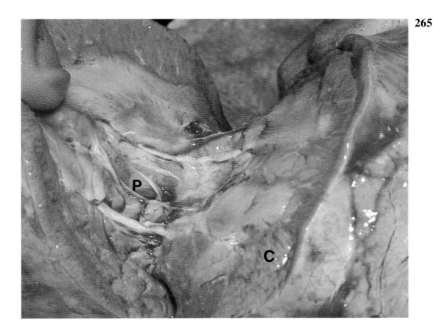

**265** Resection of a tumour in a kidney in which the kidney has been perfused with cold saline first to wash out the blood. This had made the cortex (C) pale yellow in colour. The renal pelvis (P) has been opened and can be seen in the middle of the photograph, just to the left of the midline.

The kidneys filter the blood and selectively reabsorb needed constituents. In normal function only unnecessary water and waste products are excreted. Water, urea, creatinine, uric acid and excess electrolytes, especially potassium and sulphate ions, are the main constituents of urine.

The typical extra-renal vascular anatomy consists of an anterior renal vein, and the renal artery lying in front of the pelvis, but anomalies are common and important in renal surgery, especially renal transplantation (266-273). The renal arteries are end arteries with only scanty arterial collaterals, mostly in and around the renal capsule. Thus, additional aberrant arteries always have important functions, each being responsible for its designated volume of renal parenchyma. Inferior polar vessels may be the main blood supply to the upper ureter and thus vital to the success of renal transplantation. Additional arteries may have adventitious origins from the main renal artery or may arise independently from the aorta.

Unlike the arteries, the large intra-renal veins anastomose with each other, so that ligation of an extra vein can, if necessary, be

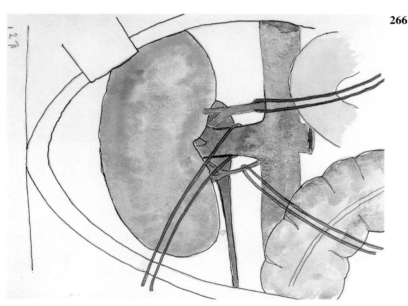

**266** Diagram of renal vessels showing two renal arteries on the right side; the lower one will be the main supply to the upper ureter. The renal vein is short on the right side.

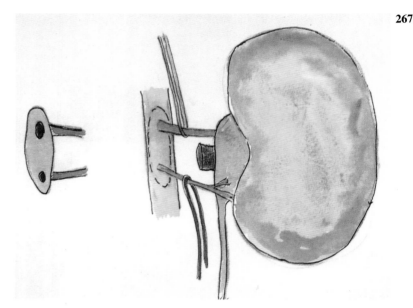

**267** Diagram of the kidney being removed for transplantation. A patch of aorta containing the orifices of the two vessels is taken so that the patch can be sewn to an incision in the recipient external iliac artery, which will not narrow the two renal vessels.

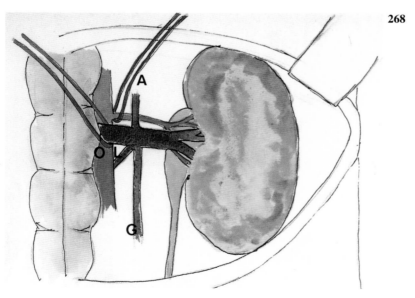

**268** Renal vessels on the left side, with slings around the renal artery and vein. The adrenal (A), gonadal (G) and a large lumbar vein (L) passing behind the aorta (O) are shown.

**269** Selective renal arteriogram with small tumour indenting the mid-portion of kidney.

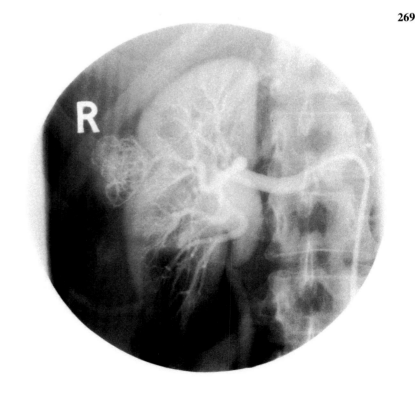

tolerated by the kidney, provided it is not the main route of venous drainage. Within the kidney, the large arterial branches divide and radiate through the parenchyma breaking up eventually into the afferent arterioles. The peritubular capillaries join to form the tributaries of the renal vein.

Both kidneys have fibrous capsules surrounding them (**274**). They are embedded in special thick condensations of perinephric fat enclosed in the fascia of Gerota* that protects them. Additional safety from trauma is provided by the lower ribs.

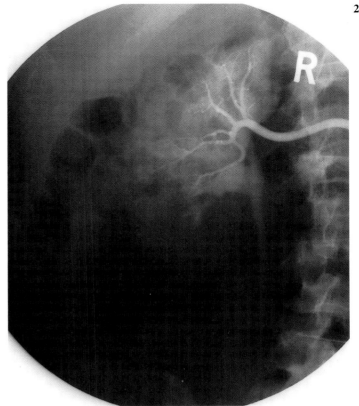

**270-272** Three separate renal arteries each supplying their own portion of kidney.

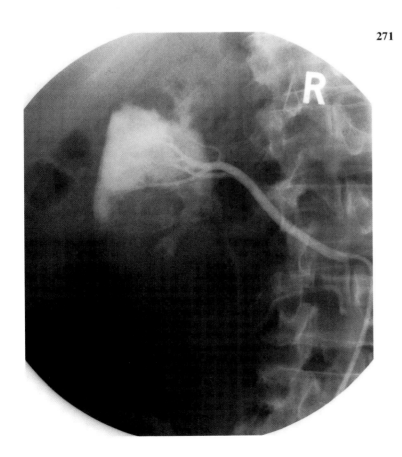

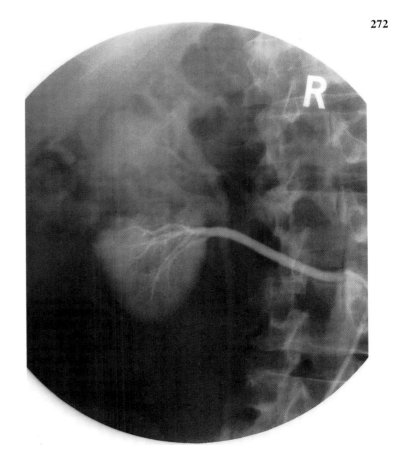

*Gerota, Dumitru (1867-1939). Professor of Surgery and Experimental Surgery – Bucharest, Rumania.

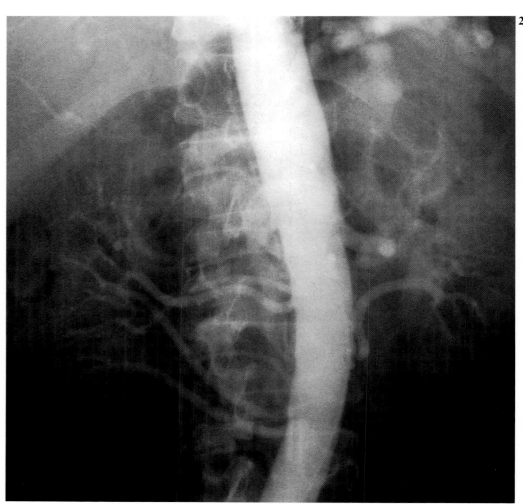

**273** Aortogram showing four renal arteries to the right kidney and two to the left kidney.

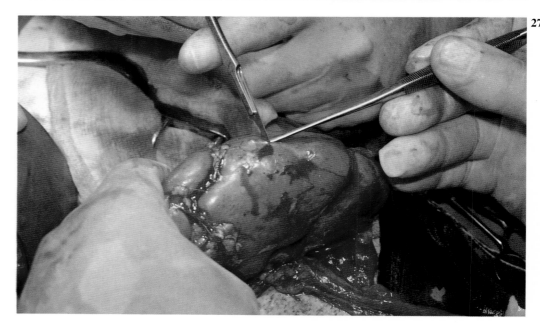

**274** Incision of the fibrous capsule of the kidney which is very delicate. The probe has been passed under the capsule and the scalpel cuts on to the probe. This is a kidney transplant.

## The Ureters

The ureters are lined, like the renal pelvis and bladder with transitional epithelium. Their courses are shown in **54** and **55** (page 28). They pass on each side beneath the posterior parietal peritoneum and in front of the psoas major muscles and lumbar vertebral transverse processes, crossing the sacro-iliac joint and passing medially to the inferior aspect of the bladder. They are supplied in their upper portions with blood from the renal vessels, in the middle third by lumbar and iliac vessels and the lowermost portion by the vesical arteries.

# The Uterus

The uterus is a midline muscular organ shaped like an inverted flask with anterior angulation, called anteversion, in relation to the vagina and flexed on itself, antiflexion. It leads to the outlet at the cervix, which is a muscular ring at the uppermost end of the stratified, squamous, epithelium lined vagina (**275-279**). The cervix is stabilized by the cardinal transverse cervical ligaments of MacKenrodt*. These ligaments are attached to the side wall of the pelvis deep to the ureters.

The vagina passes up from between the labia minora of the vulva, lying behind the urethra and bladder and in front of the anus and rectum. It passes beyond the projecting cervix resulting in a cul-de-sac ring – the vaginal fornices. The uterus is covered by visceral peritoneum. The round ligaments pass from the upper lateral extremity of the body of the uterus to the deep inguinal ring and they have the same course as the vasa deferentia in the male. They loop over the ureters and pass through the inguinal canals and out of the external ring into the labia majora of the vulva, the homologue of the scrotum.

A wide, peritoneal fold, the broad ligament leads from each side of the uterus to the side wall of the pelvis and contains in its upper free edge the fallopian tube lined with ciliated columnar epithelium, arranged in convoluted folds (**280**). This leads from the lumen of the uterus to the widened ampullary fimbriated opening of the tube adjacent to the front of the ovary; one of the fimbriae is attached to the ovary.

The uterus receives its blood supply from the uterine artery, a branch of the anterior division of the internal iliac and also from the ovarian gonadal artery, direct from the aorta. During pregnancy the uterus enlarges enormously to accommodate the developing foetus, its membranes and placenta. The blood vessels likewise enlarge to cope with these physiological needs. The ligaments of the pelvis soften to enable the birth canal to enlarge sufficiently for parturition (**282-297**).

275

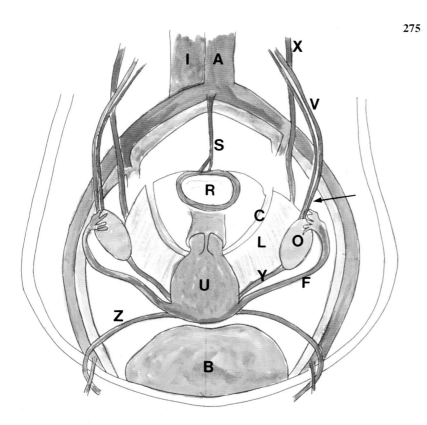

276

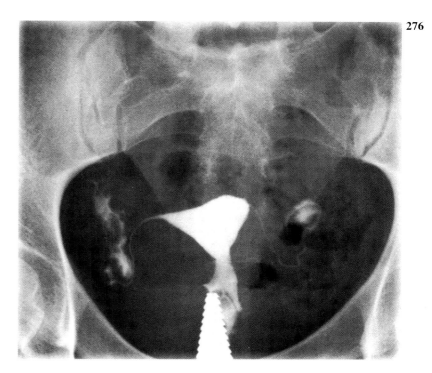

**276**   Salpingogram resulting from passing contrast per vaginum into the body of the uterus and through the fallopian tubes extending from the two horns of the uterus and into the peritoneal cavity around the ovaries.

**275**   Diagram of the female pelvis showing the bifurcation of the aorta (A), vena cava (I), and the bladder in the midline inferiorly (B). The uterus (U), with the cervix indicated, is coloured green, as are the two fallopian tubes (F). The round ligament (Z) of the uterus is indicated passing through the internal inguinal ring adjacent to the inferior epigastric artery. The ovaries (O) are seen together with their blood supply; the ovarian vessels (V) cross the ureters (X) and lying under the peritoneum pass into the top of the broad ligament as the infundibular pelvic fold (arrow) and the ovarian ligament (Y) passes from the lower pole of the ovary to the upper angle of the uterus. The broad ligament (L) of the uterus is coloured light blue. Transverse cervical ligaments of MacKenrodt are also indicated (C). Rectum (R), median sacral artery (S).

*MacKenrodt, Alwin Karl (1859-1925) Professor of Gynaecology – Berlin.

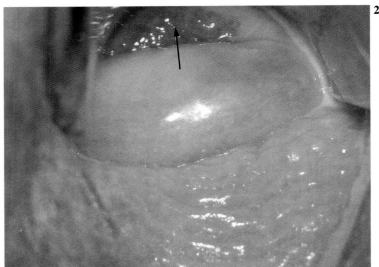

**277** A normal cervix, viewed per vaginum. The speculum in place can be seen. The red portion (arrow) in the upper central part of the photograph is the cervical columnar epithelium. The stratified squamous epithelium of the vagina and the rest of the cervix are pink in colour.

**278** Specimen of uterus and cervix removed. There is early malignant change in the mouth or os of the cervix (arrow). The forceps hold the cut edge of the vagina.

**279**

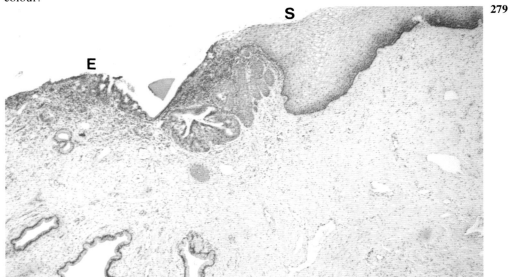

**279** Histology of the junction of the columnar cell lined endocervix (E) left, with stratified squamous lined ectocervix right (S).

**280**

**280** Histology of fallopian tube showing longitudinal folds lined by pseudostratified columnar ciliated cells.

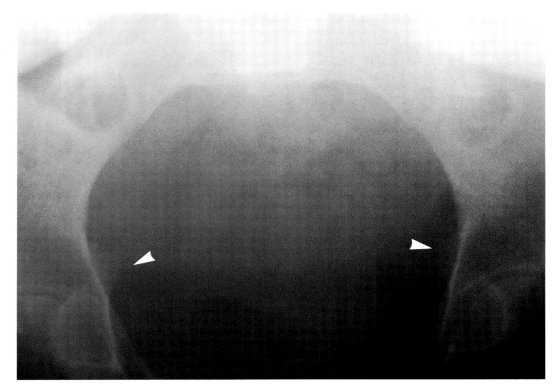

**281** X-ray of the female pelvis viewed from above, showing true pelvic inlet. The ischial spines which help in the rotation of the foetal head in mid-pelvis can also be seen (arrow heads).

**282**

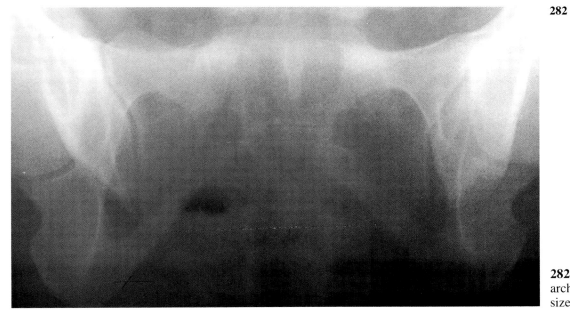

**282** X-ray of female pelvis viewed from below, showing the arch formed by the inferior pubic rami. The angle determines the size of the pelvic outlet.

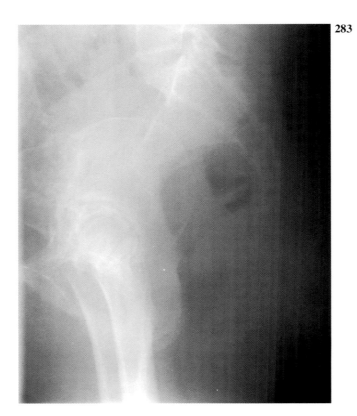

**283** Lateral X-ray of the pregnant patient; the foetal skull can be seen. More important, the dimensions of the bony pelvis can be calculated. This can be of great importance in cases where a narrow pelvis is suspected.

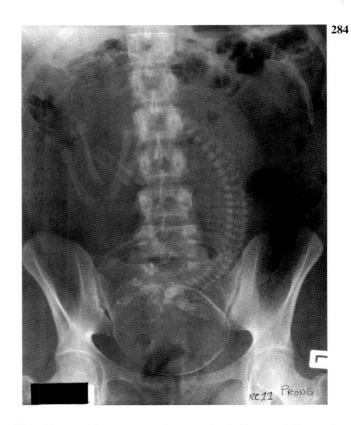

**284** X-ray of foetus at term in utero. Such films could be used to assist in assessing foetal maturity; this can now be done by ultrasound. X-rays should be avoided in pregnancy unless they are essential.

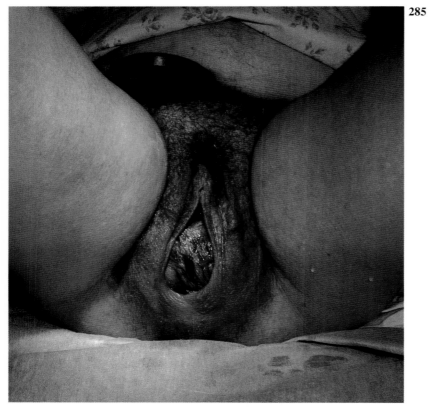

**285** The beginning of parturition. The foetal head can be seen after the cervix has dilated fully.

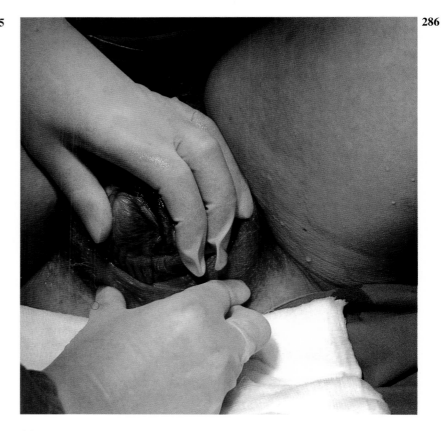

**286** The head is presenting.

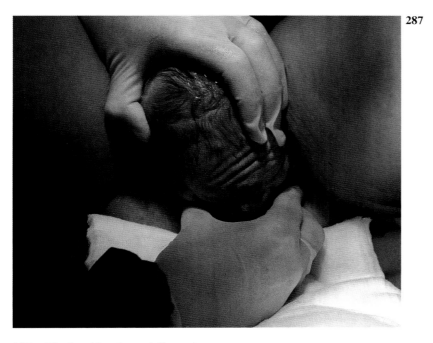

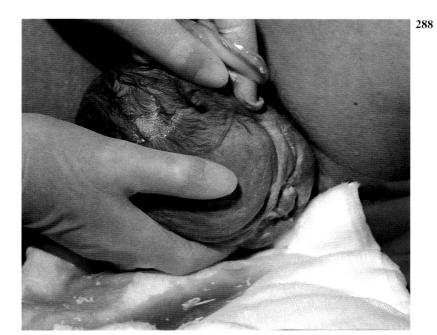

**287**  The head has been delivered.

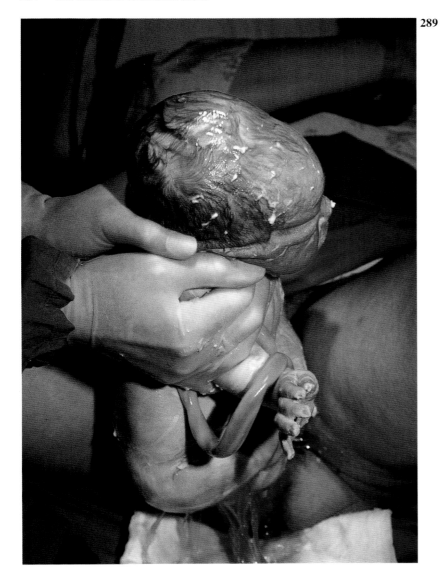

**288, 289**  Process of delivery.

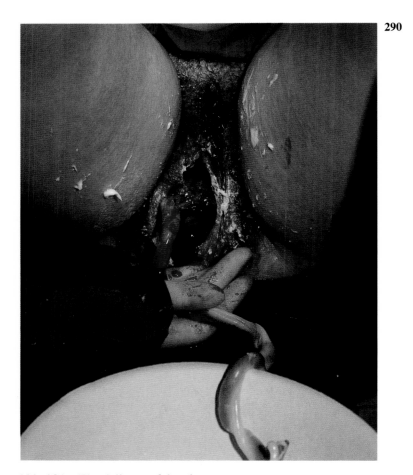

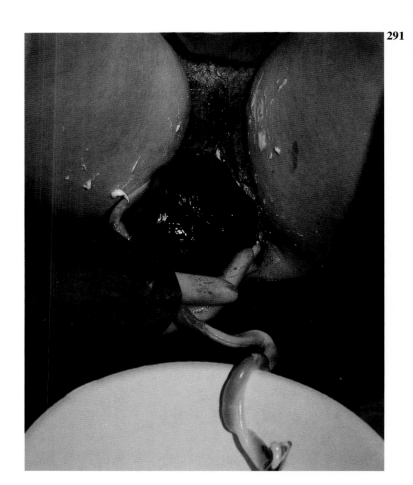

**290, 291**  The delivery of the placenta.

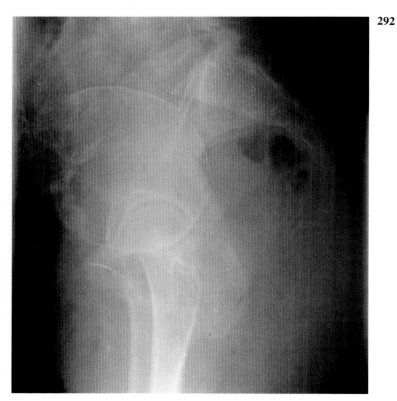

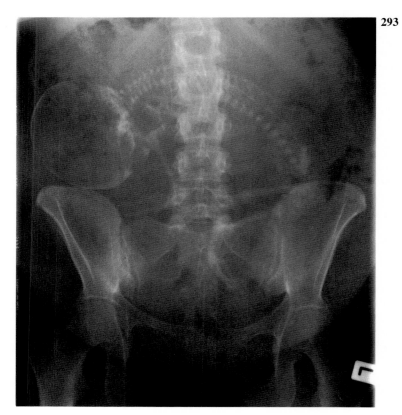

**292**  Lateral X-ray of pregnant pelvis at term. The head is not quite engaged.

**293**  X-ray of the pelvis at term showing transverse lie with the head under the mother's right costal margin and the breech in the left iliac fossa.

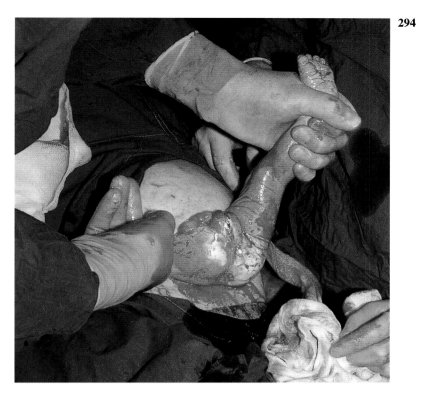

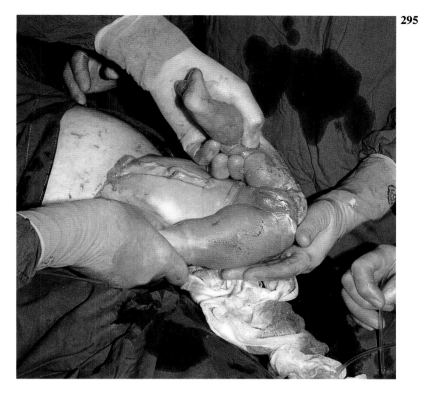

**294** Caesarian section through a lower abdominal incision. The uterus is approached, the child presenting as a breech is delivered.

**295** Delivery nearly completed.

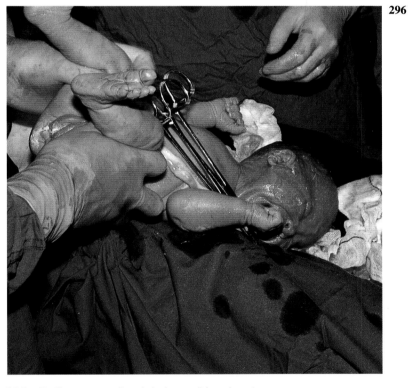

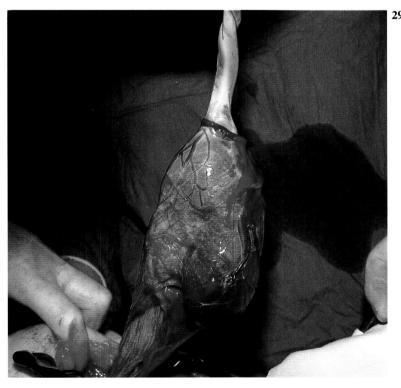

**296** Delivery completed, baby sucking thumb.

**297** Removal of the placenta.

# The Ovaries

These 3 x 2 cm oval organs lie close to the side wall of the pelvis behind the ends of the fallopian tubes. They are attached by peritoneum overlying the ovarian vessels passing from the pelvic side wall in the infundibulo-pelvic ligament and another peritoneal fold, the *mesovarium*, to the posterior layer of the broad ligament. The *ovarian ligament* is a fibrous band passing from the lower pole of the ovary to the upper angle of the uterus and continues as the round ligament. The ovaries are sited so that ova, liberated freely into the peritoneal cavity from the rupture of the Graafian follicles each month (**298**), pass naturally into the tube which is lined by ciliated columnar epithelium and do not wander around the peritoneal cavity. Fertilization occurs in the fallopian tube. The cilia propel the fertilized egg into the cavity of the uterus. The zygote becomes embedded in the uterine lining of endometrium where embryonic development takes place. A fertilized ovum may develop ectopically in the fallopian tube. An ectopic pregnancy can present as a surgical emergency with exsanguinating intraperitoneal haemorrhage usually 6 weeks after the last normal period.

The proximity of the cervix, uterine and ovarian arteries and round ligament to the ureter puts this vital urinary drainage duct in danger during removal of the ovary, uterus and in many other pelvic operations. It is safest to deliberately dissect out the ureter, identify it by its writhing vermiculations and put a soft rubber sling around it so that it is not damaged (**299, 300**). A cut ureter will leak urine during the operation (**301**), an error that may be instantly recognized and rectified by end-to-end suture over a stent. If not recognized during operation, urinary ascites post-operatively can cause the patient much morbidity.

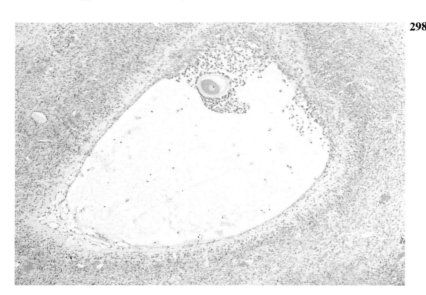

**298**  Histology of ovary showing a Graafian follicle.

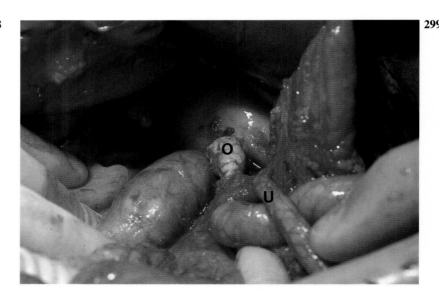

**299**  The pelvis looked at from above. In the middle, coloured white, there is a cobblestone appearance of the ovary (O). The ureter (U) is passing under the surgeon's thumb very close to the ovary.

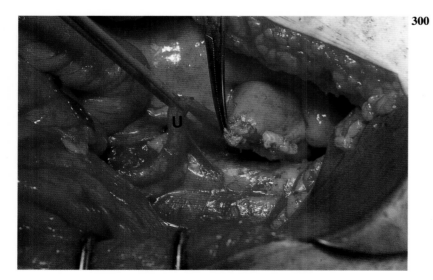

**300**  The ureter (U) has been protected by passing a sling around it so it will not be damaged. Forceps are applied to the fallopian tube which has been divided where it joins the uterus. The ovary and fallopian tube have been removed.

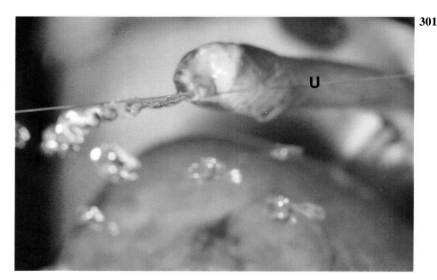

**301**  The ureter (U) is producing urine; this is a case for renal transplant. The ureter has not yet been implanted in the bladder.

# The Bladder

This is a muscular hollow organ lined by highly specialized urine resistant transitional epithelium (**302**). When contracted, the lumen is obliterated unless there is a urinary obstruction. The relatively fixed base of the bladder is a triangular portion called the trigone, with the urethra opening below. At the other angles of the trigone the ureters enter (**303-308**). They pass through the bladder wall obliquely, the distal portion lying under the bladder mucosa so that when the intravesical pressure rises in voiding, the mucosa is pressed against the terminal ureter, effectively occluding its lumen. This valve action is of great importance. If defective, urine is expelled back into the ureter and renal pelvis during micturition, leading to dilatation of the ureters, back pressure on the kidneys and impaired renal function (**309-311**).

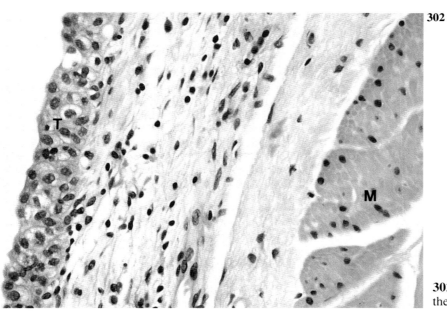

**302**

**302** Histology of the ureter shows the smooth muscle (M) on the right and the transitional epithelium on the left (T).

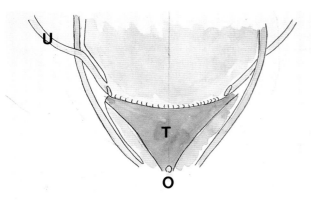

**303**

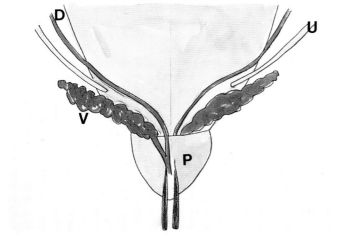

**303** Above: Diagram of the trigone of the bladder. On the left hand side can be seen the arrangement of the ureter (U) passing through the muscle wall of the bladder and under the mucosa. When the bladder fills, the intravesical pressure forces the walls of the ureter together, preventing reflux of urine. This is the normal sphincteric mechanism. The trigone (T) is seen between the two ureters with the urethral orifice in the middle inferiorly (O).

Below: diagram of male pelvis viewed from behind. The ureter (U) can be seen entering the bladder. The vas deferens (D) passes on the posterior surface of the bladder where it joins the drainage duct of the seminal vesicles (V) which pass through the prostate (P).

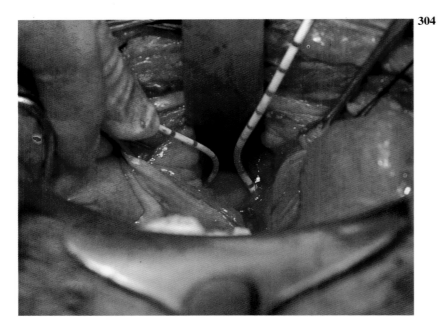

**304** Two catheters inserted at open operation into the ureteric orifices, through the lumen of the bladder.

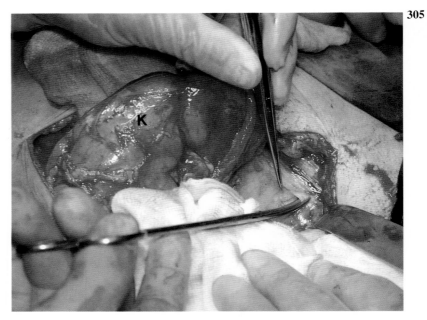

**305** Dissection of the bladder in a kidney transplant operation. The kidney (K) has been vascularized but the ureter has not yet been implanted.

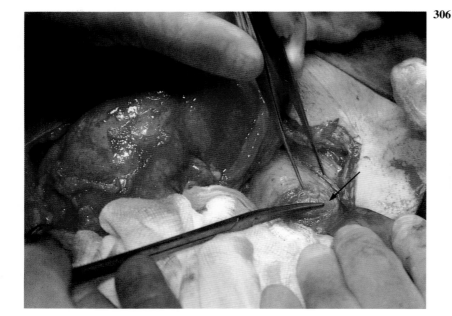

**306** Continuation of the dissection of the muscle of the bladder wall. The bladder mucosa is beginning to show as a bluish bulge (arrow).

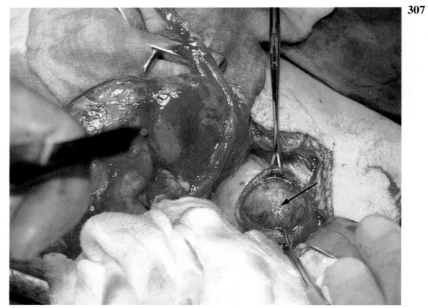

**307** The bladder mucosa is now pouting out (arrow).

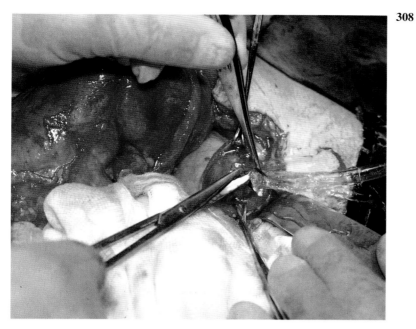

**308** The mucosa has been incised for implantation of the ureter. The urine contained in the bladder is escaping and is being aspirated through a sucker.

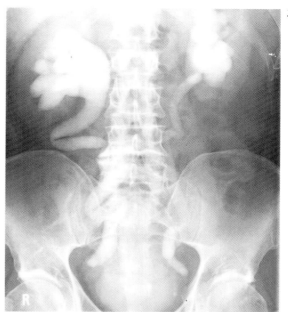

**309** A patient with prostatic obstruction and back pressure effects on ureters and pelvicalyceal system, producing marked distension.

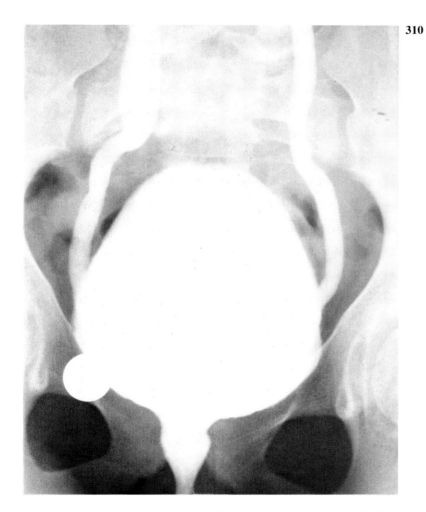

**310** A child with vesico-ureteric reflux. Contrast has been instilled into the bladder through a catheter and the patient has been asked to micturate. Contrast passes up the ureters.

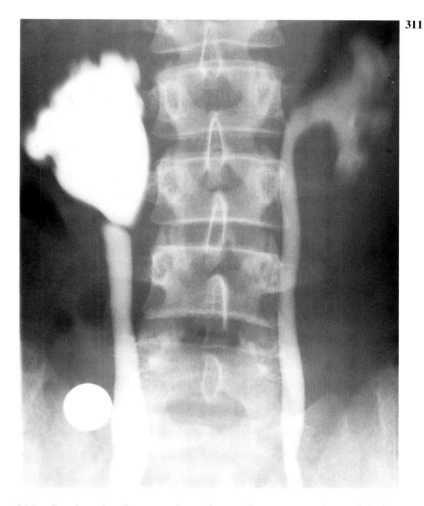

**311** Continuation from previous picture: the upper renal tract is being distended due to reflux.

# The Male Urethra and Prostate

The urethra passes from the inferior apex of the trigone of the bladder down through the prostate. At the base of the bladder the smooth muscle continues to surround the origin of the urethra as the *internal sphincter*, innervated by the autonomic system, and like the internal sphincter of the anus, it is not under full voluntary control (**312**). The prostate, composed of glandular and fibrous tissue, not unlike the breast histologically, (**313, 314**) surrounds the urethra. Its numerous ducts open into the posterior urethral wall. In a young man the prostate is about the size of a chestnut, 4 x 3 cm, orientated with its apex pointing down. There are two lateral lobes with a median sulcus posteriorly.

Above the entrance of the ejaculatory ducts is the pyramidal shaped middle or median lobe, which often projects into the bladder in old age. When enlarged, the prostate elongates the contained urethra, which may develop a circuitous path. The upper posterior portion enlarges as a pathological median lobe, which interferes with the function of the internal sphincter. This widens the outflow of the bladder into the urethra and allows urine to be in contact with the posterior urethra, even when the bladder is relatively empty. This gives an urgent desire to micturate, worse when the patient lies in bed at night. So there is frequency of micturition, especially nocturnal. The elongated tortuous urethra becomes partially obstructed, so in order to void urine, the bladder hypertrophies and the enlarged smooth muscle bands form trabeculae which can be seen cystoscopically and on cystograms (**315-317**). Between these the transitional epithelium of the bladder mucosa may be pushed out as a diverticulum, which fills with urine during contraction of the bladder and empties during bladder relaxation giving the symptoms of double micturition or "pis à deux". (**318, 319**).

**312**

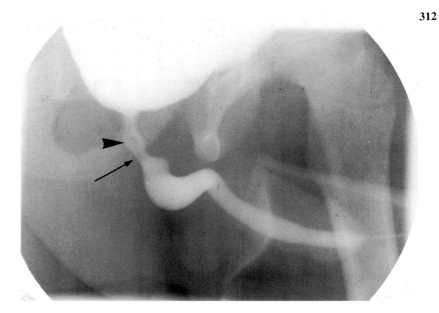

**312** A normal male cysto-urethrogram. Contrast medium previously instilled into the bladder. During micturition the whole length of the urethra is visible. The prostatic urethra is recognized by the impression of the verumontanum (arrow head) which marks the point of entry of the ejaculatory ducts. Just distal to this there is the narrower membranous urethra (arrow). Bulbous and penile urethra more distally.

**313**

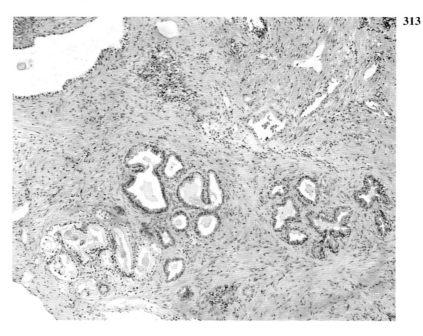

**313** Histology of the prostate with glandular epithelium arranged in acini, between which are smooth muscle and collagen fibres.

**314**

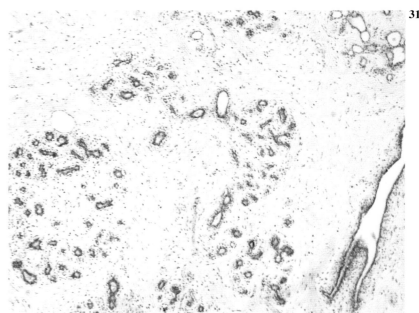

**314** Histology of the breast. Similar to the prostate but there is no smooth muscle.

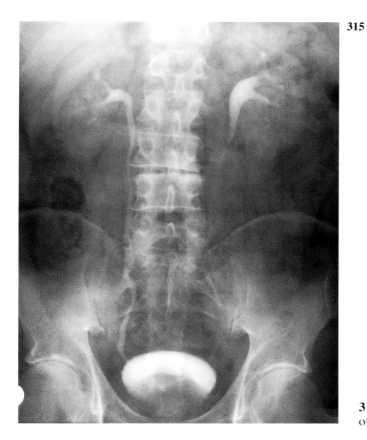

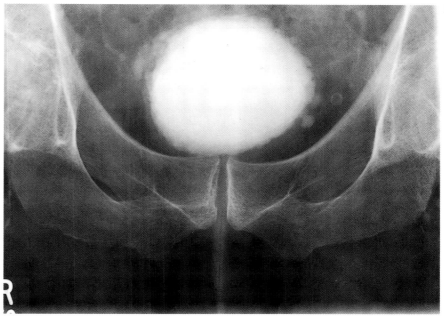

**316** Another patient with prostatic obstruction in whom the bladder outline is uneven due to trabeculation caused by hypertrophy of the muscle in the bladder wall.

**315** Patient with prostatic hypertrophy in whom an IVU shows a large prostatic indentation of the base of the bladder.

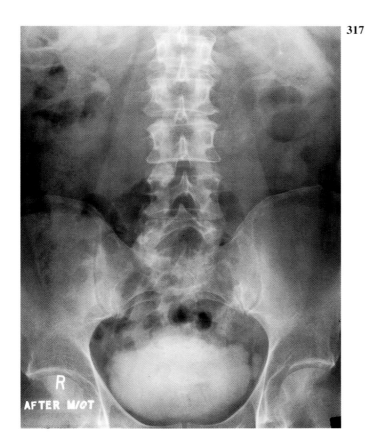

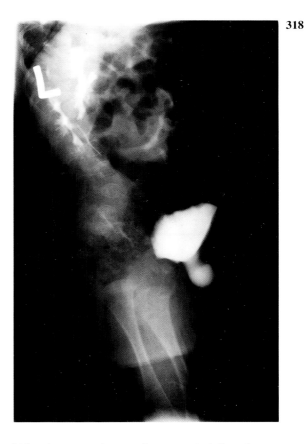

**317** Another patient with prostatic hypertrophy. IVU film obtained after the patient has passed urine: there is still a large residuum of contrast in the bladder which cannot be completely emptied.

**318** An unusual case of a congenital diverticulum of the bladder.

The joint ejaculatory ducts from the seminal vesicles and vasa deferentia open into the prostatic urethra beside a posterior running ridge, the *urethral crest* or verumontanum (**320**). Having passed through the prostate the urethra pierces the perineal membrane, becoming the short and relatively narrow membranous portion with its intrinsic external sphincter mechanism (see page 54). The urethra then enters the bulb which is surrounded by the bulbo-spongiosus muscle innervated by the perineal branch of the pudendal nerve (S2,3 and 4). The urethra within the corpus spongiosum of the penis leads to the external urethral orifice. This portion of the urethra is the common site for an inflammatory stricture, typically post gonococcal. An enlarged prostate removed by open or closed endoscopic surgery destroys the internal urinary sphincter at the base of the bladder, causing the patient to ejaculate into the bladder instead of externally.

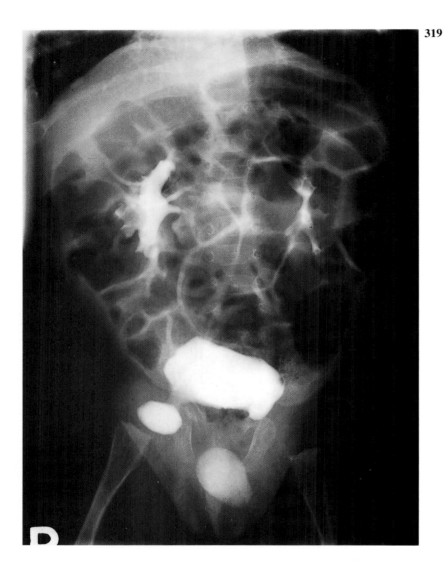

**319**    Continuation from previous picture: the diverticulum is shown to be passing into an inguinal hernia through the internal inguinal ring.

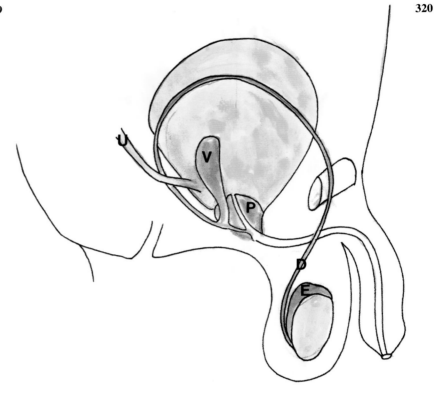

**320**    Diagram of the vas deferens (D) leaving the epididymis (E), passing through the inguinal canal, looping over the ureter (U) and joining behind the prostate (P) the seminal vesicle (V) and then opening into the prostatic urethra at the verumontanum.

# The Lumbar Sympathetic Chain

On each side on the front of the bodies of the lumbar vertebrae along the medial margins of the psoas muscles lie the right and left sympathetic chains, which can be identified by a finger tip rolling over them. At each segment is a ganglion (**321-323**). The white rami pass from the lower thoracic T6-12 and first two lumbar segments. The four lumbar ganglia are relay centres, from which grey postganglionic sympathetic branches pass to the viscera via segmental nerves and especially along arteries.

The sympathetic chain passes over the promontory of the sacrum to form the hypogastric plexus which communicates via branches called the *presacral nerves* with parasympathetic fibres from the sacral plexus, S2, 3 and 4, called the pelvic splanchnic nerves. These innervate the bladder, rectum and uterus and their nervi erigentes branches are vaso-dilator to the erectile tissue of the external genitalia. The sympathetic chains join in the midline in front of the coccyx in a single *ganglion impar*. Sensory nerves follow the autonomic nerves. If the sympathetic chain is removed, vasomotor tone in the legs is abolished. If both L1 ganglia are removed the mechanism of ejaculation is lost. Damage to the parasympathetic nervi erigentes will prevent erection of the external genitalia.

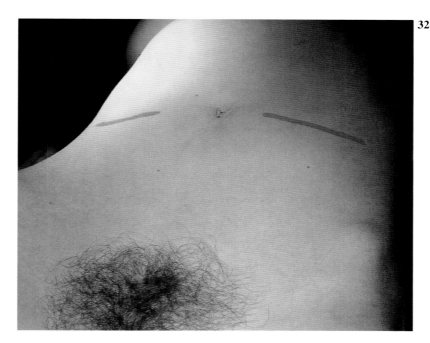

**321** Patient prepared for a lumbar sympathectomy. Short incisions are made one each side at the level of the umbilicus. The peritoneum is pushed away and the lumbar sympathetic chains are found on the front of the bodies of the lumbar vertebrae at the medial edge of each psoas muscle.

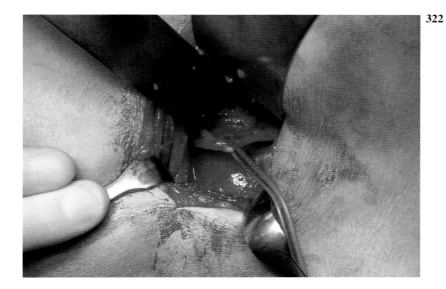

**322** A sling has been passed around the sympathetic chain and a ganglion can be seen.

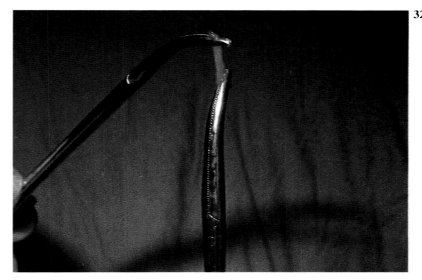

**323** The lumbar sympathetic chain is fairly tough and will support the weight of heavy forceps as shown in the photograph.

# The Thoracic Duct

This narrow conduit arises from the cisterna chyli lymph sac which is situated in front of L1 and 2 bodies under the right crus of the diaphragm. It collects lymph from the lower limbs and all the abdominal viscera (**324, 325**). If cut the leakage of lymph will be white in colour due to the fat content of the small intestinal lymph called chyle, which is absorbed directly without digestion. The lymphatic vessels in the intestinal wall and mesentery are called lacteals due to the white appearance resembling milk. The thoracic duct passes into the chest behind and to the right of the aorta. It reaches the back of the oesophagus and passes to the left, and ends by reaching the neck through the thoracic inlet and joining the left subclavian vein close to its junction with the internal jugular vein.

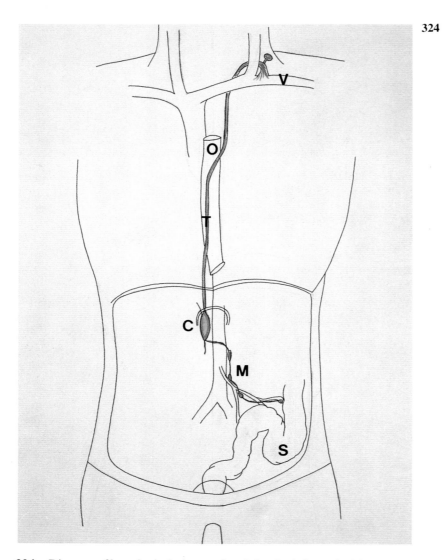

324

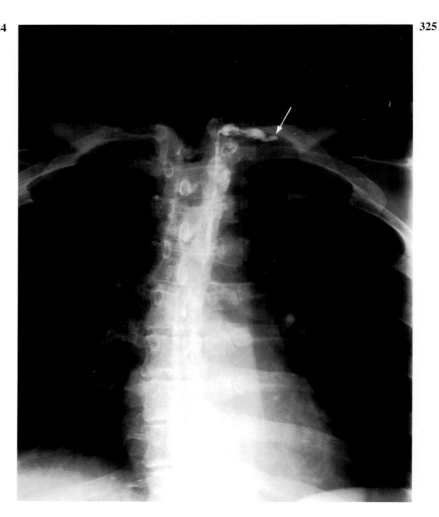

325

**325** Lymphangiogram showing the termination of the thoracic duct in the neck, where it passes into the left subclavian vein (arrow).

**324** Diagram of lymphatic drainage of an abdominal viscus; in this case, the sigmoid colon (S). Lymphatics drain into lymph nodes adjacent to the viscus and then pass into lymph nodes in the sigmoid mesocolon (M) and from there into pre-aortic lymph nodes and para-aortic lymph nodes. From the whole abdomen lymphatic drainage is collected in the large lymphatic sac, the cisterna chyli (C) to the right of the aorta. This is drained by the long thoracic duct (T) which passes through the aortic orifice in the diaphragm deep to the median arcuate ligament to behind the oesophagus (O) where it crosses from the right to the left side, passes through the thoracic inlet and enters the subclavian vein (V), usually adjacent to the jugular vein.

Other lymph nodes drain at this point and retrograde permeation of tumour into lymph nodes in the left supraclavicular fossa may be a sign of cancer in the abdomen.

# 5 Some Symptoms and Signs of Deranged Anatomy

The previous chapters on visceral topography and the structure of the abdominal wall and the abdominal organs should provide a framework that will allow some common examples of deranged anatomy to be explained.

## General Considerations

Listening to the patient's story carefully, paying especial attention to the time of onset, sequence and course of the symptoms will often point directly to the diagnosis. Any attempt to distort the history to make it fit a diagnosis is more likely to lead the clinician astray.

Careful physical examination, going deliberately through the stages of inspection, palpation, percussion and auscultation is much more likely to be rewarded with the correct diagnosis, than an instant "snap diagnosis" based on "experience" which has been cynically described as "making the same mistake repeatedly with increasing confidence".

Lord Brock*, a very great clinical teacher, would point out to his students: "The first and greatest step towards establishing a surgical diagnosis is to determine exactly in which anatomical site the lesion lies, then to consider the most likely pathological explanation for the findings." Of course, to do this a knowledge of anatomy is essential! The possibilities can be listed in order of preference, as a bookmaker will list the odds of runners in a race. Instead of previous form, the reputation of the jockey and weather conditions, the surgeon must take note of how common the condition is, the age and sex of the patient, any special factors in family history, occupation, habits, previous medical history, how ill the patient is, how reliable the history, physical signs and any special investigations. If everything points to a rare lesion, for example, a *psoas abscess*, there is no virtue in sticking to the diagnosis of an inguinal hernia. "If you see an elephant walking down Oxford Street†, accept it as such. It would be foolish to call it a bus just because buses are more commonly seen in that situation."

The surgical sieve is a useful prop if there are difficulties. Could the lesion best be explained as congenital, traumatic, infective, malignant, degenerative, metabolic or (increasingly as medical management becomes more complicated) iatrogenic?

## Pain

This is the commonest and usually the most distressing of symptoms. In the abdomen, pain is discretely experienced as emanating from the somatic sensory nerves of the skin, abdominal wall and parietal peritoneum. Internal viscera, when damaged, do not emit a localized pain and hollow viscera only become painful if their outlets are blocked or blood supply impaired. The pain due to distension of a hollow viscus with a smooth muscle wall is referred to the location of neural somatic segmental supply from which their autonomic nerves are derived. The oesophagus, stomach, proximal duodenum, pan-

creas, liver, gall bladder and spleen are all foregut embryological midline organs. Pain will be referred to the epigastrium T8 and 9 (**326**). If the parietal peritoneum is irritated by blood, for example from a ruptured spleen, or pus from an inflamed appendix, then pain will be experienced from the corresponding segment of parietal peritoneum; left hypochondrium or right iliac fossa in the examples given. Irritation of the parietal peritoneum lining the diaphragm will cause pain referred to the corresponding shoulder (**327**).

Pain referred from the midgut, from mid duodenum to the splenic flexure of the colon, is felt in the periumbilical region T10-11. Pain from the hindgut, descending and pelvic colon, rectum, bladder and uterus is felt suprapubically in the hypogastrium, T12-L1. The laterally derived organs, adrenals, kidneys, ureters and gonads will have pain referred to the same side often extending in the oblique distribution of the segmental nerves. Adrenal and renal pains are felt in the loin extending forward to T11, renal pelvic, ureter T12, and gonads L1.

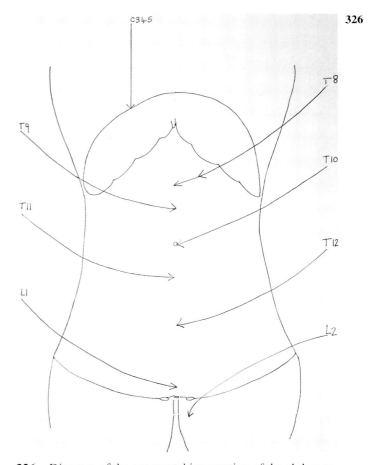

**326**

**326** Diagram of the segmental innervation of the abdomen.

*Brock, Russell Claude (1903-1980). Surgeon, Guy's Hospital, London.
†Equivalent to Madison Avenue.

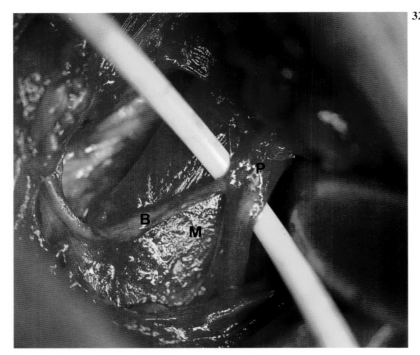

Pain may be of sudden onset, "like a knife", with the patient lying still to prevent exacerbation – e.g. a perforated viscus; or throbbing exacerbated by each heart beat, e.g. an abscess; or colicky with dreadful exacerbations where the patient feels that something is twisting inside him. He will tend to writhe about during the spasms and vomit due to the pain. Colic occurs with obstruction of bowel, ureter, bladder, uterus or gall bladder; all of which are hollow organs with smooth muscle walls.

**327** Photograph of a section of the phrenic (P) nerve in the neck overlying the scalenus anterior muscle (M). In this case a branch (B) can be seen passing to supply the supraclavicular region, explaining the relationship of referred pain from the diaphragm to the shoulder tip.

## Swelling

A common presentation of surgical outpatients is a lump in the abdomen or groin. It is first necessary to be sure that the lump originates from within the abdomen and not within or superficial to the abdominal wall. If the patient tenses the anterior abdominal muscles by lifting up his head and legs, a superficial lump will become more prominent, a deep lesion will disappear. Thus an undescended testis in the inguinal canal will become impalpable, whilst a testis ectopic in the superficial inguinal pouch, a much more common abnormality, will be felt easily (**328-330**).

The lesion should be palpated with the hand kept still to detect pulsation. It is surprising how often a poor clinician will keep his hands in motion, as if he has an uncontrollable tic, and completely miss the expansile pulsation in an aneurysm. Then without touching the lump the patient is asked to cough. If the lump has a cough impulse this is most likely to be a hernia but may be a sapheno-varix or a psoas abscess. A hernia is reducible, a sapheno-varix can be emptied and felt to fill and will transmit a thrill if the saphenous vein below is tapped. A hernia may not have a visible cough impulse, but one may be detected on gentle palpation with the hand kept *still*. A psoas abscess can extend above and below the inguinal ligament. Pressure above will be appreciated by palpation below and vice versa – cross fluctuation (**331-333**).

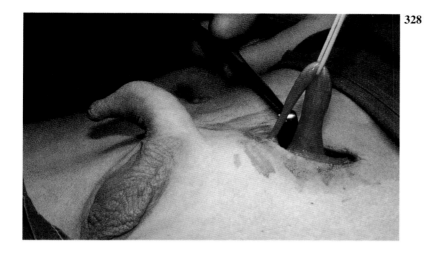

**328**

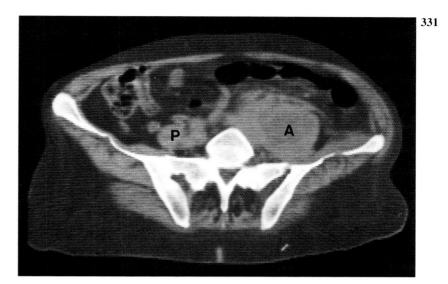

**331**

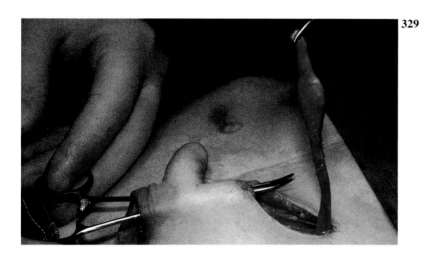

**329**

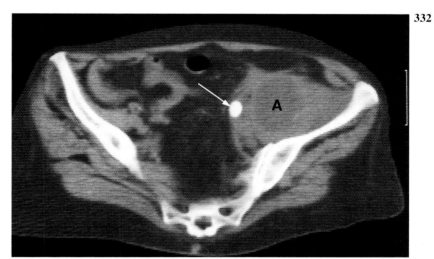

**332**

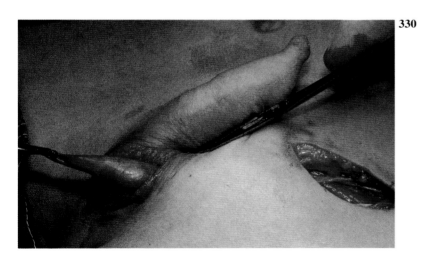

**330**

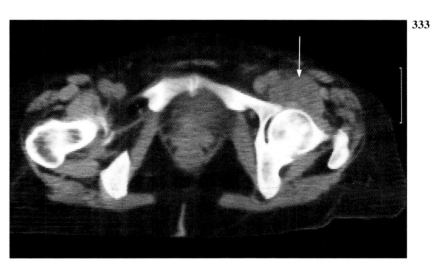

**333**

**328–330** Stages in operative treatment of an ectopic testis. The groin incision was over the testis in the superficial inguinal pouch, the cord being mobilized and then the testis brought down to the base of the scrotum where it is fixed.

**331 – 333** A series of CT images in an elderly patient with septicaemia and hip pain. A large left psoas abscess (A) is shown; compare with the normal psoas (P) on the right in **331**. In **332** a large ureteric calculus is shown (arrow); infection of the left kidney and ureter was the predisposing cause of the psoas abscess in this patient. In **333** the caudal extent of the enlarged psoas is seen presenting (arrow) caudal to the inguinal ligament.

A swelling in the scrotum may be a hernia, in which case one cannot get above it on palpation. True scrotal swellings, e.g. of testis, hydrocoele, epididymal cyst, are confined to the scrotum. One can palpate their upper limit.

Hydrocoeles and epididymal cysts are fluctuant and usually transilluminate brilliantly. A hydrocoele surrounds the testis, which may therefore be difficult to feel as it lies posterior in the distended tunica vaginalis (**334-337**). An epididymal cyst lies behind and above and can be moved separately from the testis (**338-341**). A hernia may be fixed or incarcerated with the neck of the sac occluded. This is a

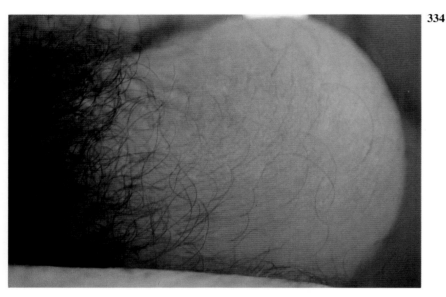

**334** Trans-illumination of a hydrocoele. The light placed behind the scrotum shows general trans-illumination, indicating the presence of clear fluid in the hydrocoele.

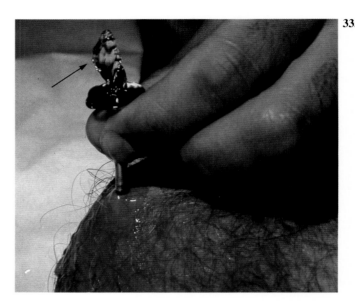

**335** Drainage of clear fluid (arrow) from the hydrocoele sac.

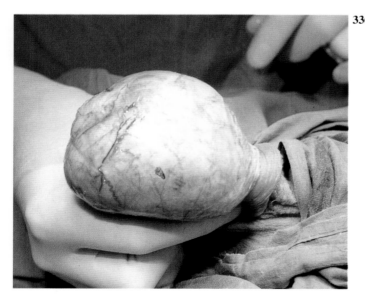

**336** Operation for hydrocoele. Scrotal incision; the tunica vaginalis is exposed.

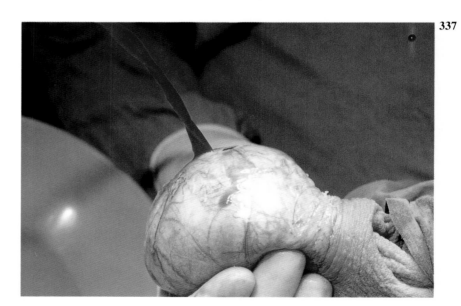

**337** At operation there was blood-stained fluid in the hydrocoele sac, the result of drainage.

common finding with a femoral hernia, which may be impossible to differentiate from an enlarged node of Cloquet in the femoral canal on clinical examination. The patient should always be examined standing after he has been examined in the recumbent position, since some swellings, particularly herniae and saphenovarices are more clearly demonstrated in the upright posture (**342**).

A true nonpulsatile intra-abdominal mass may be an enlarged diseased organ or an adventitious swelling such as an appendix abscess. The simple physical characteristics that are typically found in enlarged organs are as follows.

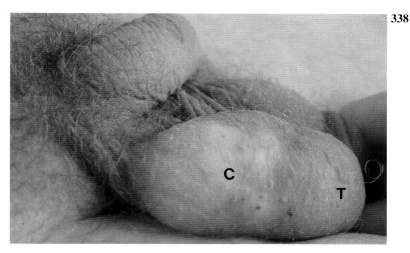

**338**  Trans-illumination of the scrotum in the case of an epididymal cyst. Testis (T), cyst (C).

**339-341**  Operation on the epididymal cyst. In **341** the testis (T) is in the surgeon's hand. The relationship of the cyst (C) to the testis can be seen.

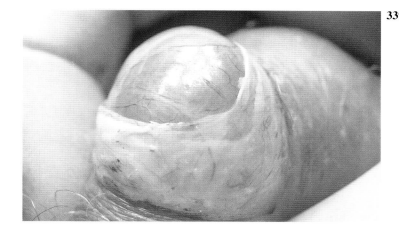

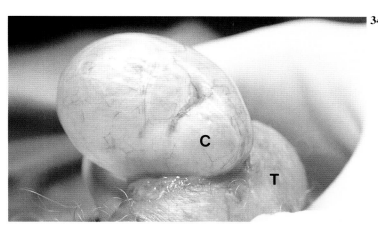

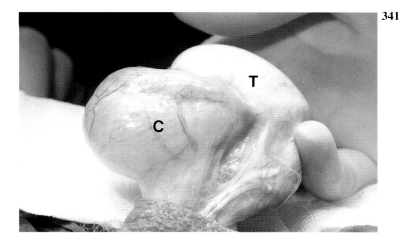

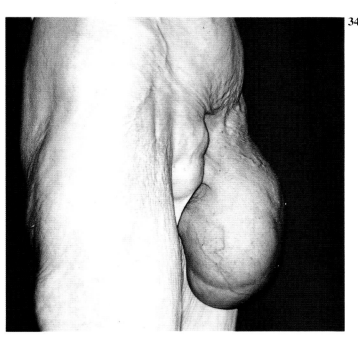

**342**  A female patient with bilateral recurrent femoral hernias demonstrated most clearly when she stands. The one of the left side is huge.

# Liver

Swelling below the right costal margin, moves with respiration. Has an edge below which the fingers can dip, dull to percussion. The hand cannot be passed above it (**343-354**).

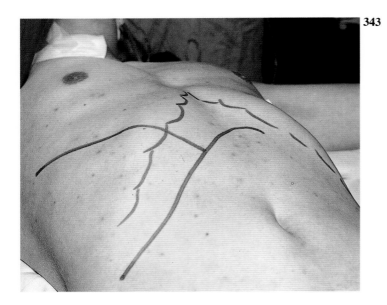

**343** A patient with hepatomegaly due to a tumour of the liver. The markings show the costal margin and the proposed sub-costal incision with extension into the eighth intercostal space.

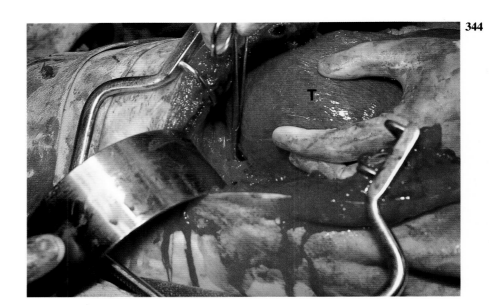

**344** Operation of case shown in **343**: the tumour (T) in the right lobe of the liver is displayed.

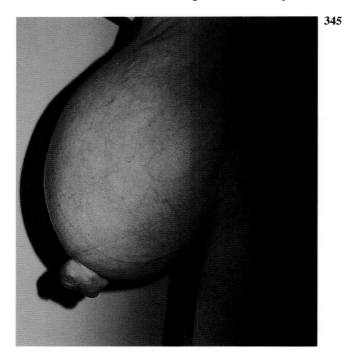

**345** A patient with enormous ascites due to a polycystic liver. There is also a parumbilical hernia at the tip of the ascites.

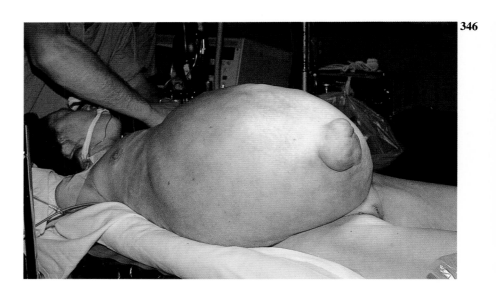

**346** The patient prepared for operation.

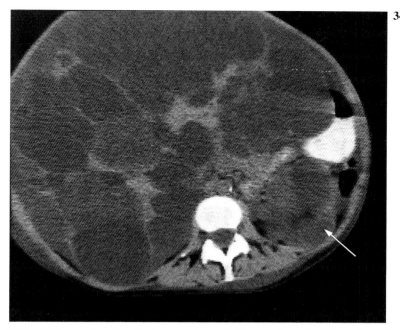

**347** CT scan showing the huge polycystic liver and moderately enlarged polycystic left kidney (arrow).

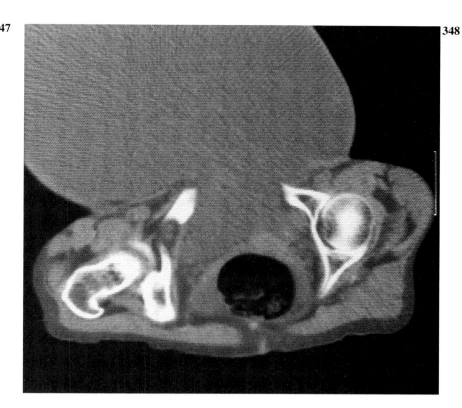

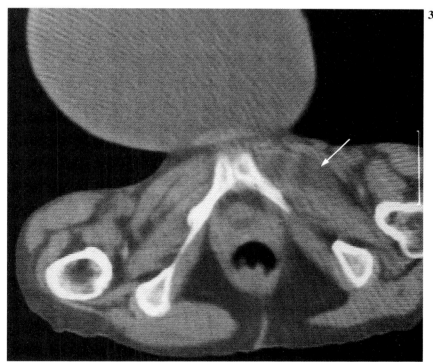

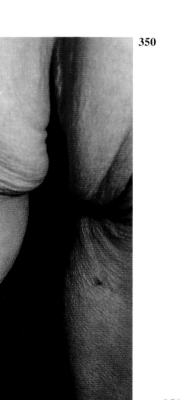

**350** The patient also had a fluctuant swelling (S) with a cough impulse in the medial side of the left thigh posteriorly. This became prominent when she stood up.

**348, 349** CT scan showing the ascitic abdominal contents protruding from the front of the abdomen. In **349** the hernia can just be seen (arrow) between the obturator externus and pectineus muscles.

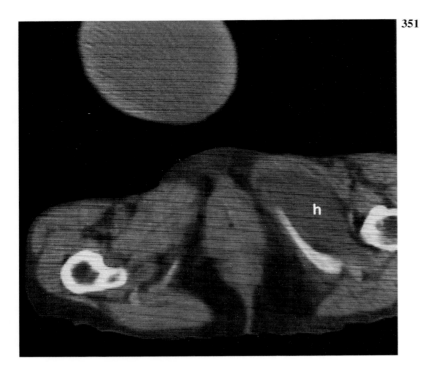

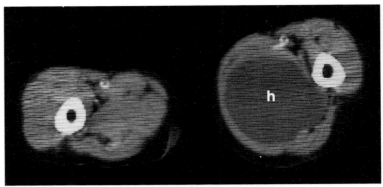

**351, 352** CT images show this to be an obturator hernia (h) extending through the obturator foramen and posteriorly into the thigh.

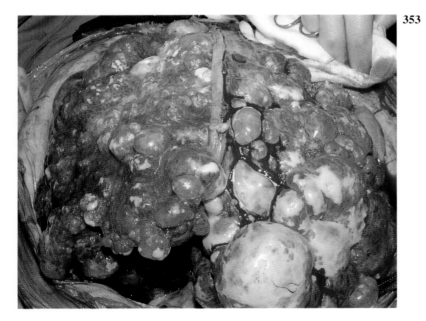

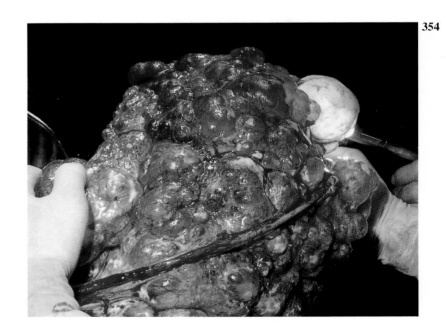

**353, 354** Photographs of the polycystic liver at operation. In **354** one of the cysts has been trans-illuminated.

# Gall Bladder

A pear shaped swelling below the right costal margin usually moves with and in continuity with the liver (**355, 356**). A large gall bladder in the presence of obstructive jaundice is unlikely to be due to stones, since they usually cause fibrosis and contraction of the gall bladder (Courvoisier's* Law).

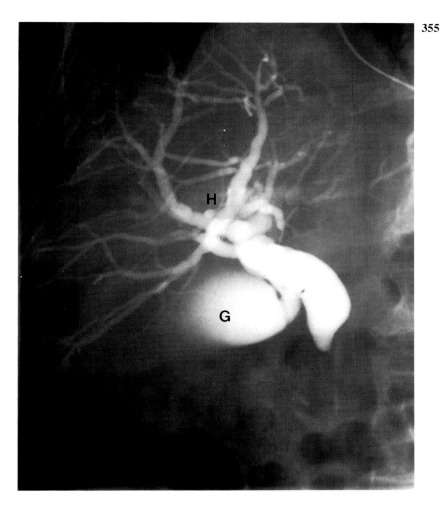

**355** A transhepatic cholangiogram in a case of carcinoma of the head of the pancreas obstructing the common bile duct and causing gross dilatation of the hepatic ducts (H) and enlargement of the gall bladder (G).

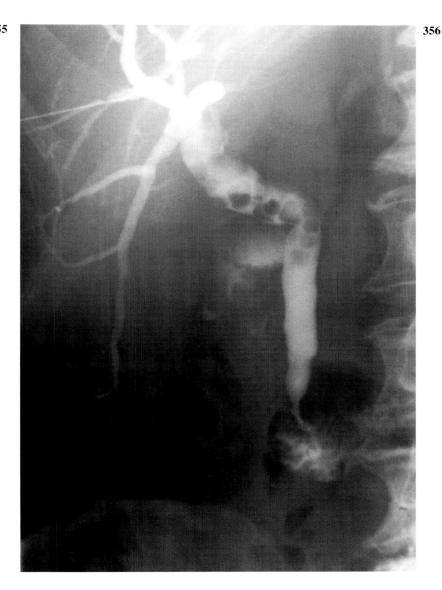

**356** A trans-hepatic cholangiogram in a patient with multiple gall stones, in this case causing blockage of the biliary system. The gall bladder is small: Courvoisier's Law.

*Courvoisier, Ludwig Georg (1843-1918) Professor of Surgery – Basle.

# Spleen

A swelling below the left costal margin, if exceptionally enlarged, may extend to the right iliac fossa. Moves with respiration and can be pushed forwards and ballotted with the left hand pressing forwards in the upper loin, especially if the patient is turned partially on to the right side with the right hand palpating in front. It is dull to percussion and the oft remembered notch can seldom be felt. The hand cannot be passed above it (**357-363**).

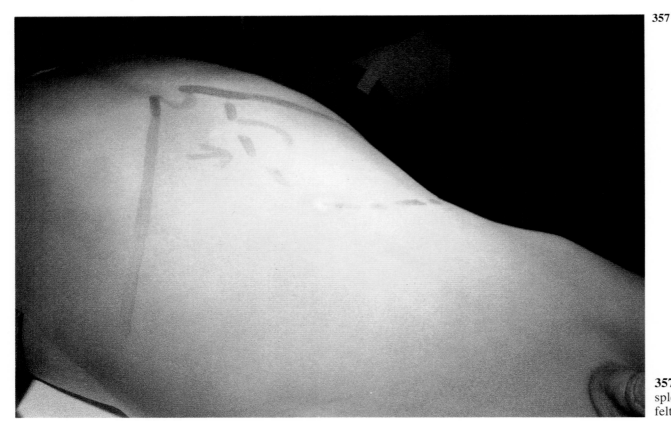

**357**

**357** Markings on a patient with splenomegaly. A medical student felt the notch and marked it.

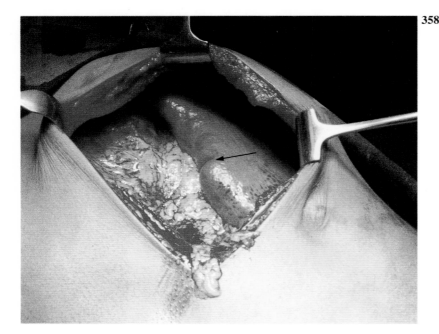

**358**

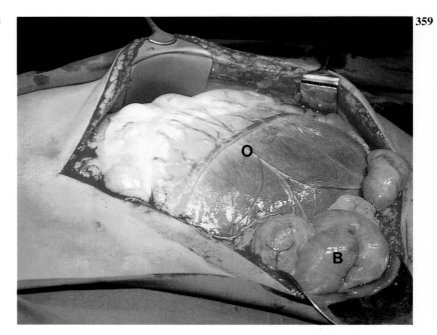

**359**

**358** At laparotomy the position of marking the notch (arrow) was exactly correct.

**359** A patient with an enormous spleen, suffering from myelosclerosis. The spleen is covered with omentum (O). Small bowel (B).

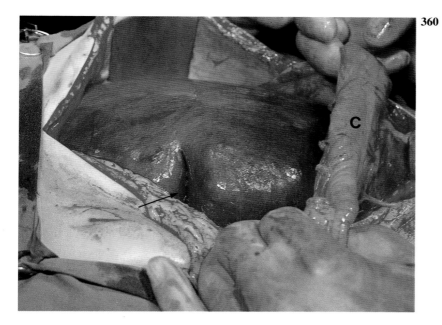

**360** Mobilization of the spleen. The notch (arrow) can be seen. The splenic flexure of the colon (C) has been separated from the greater curve of the stomach and the phrenico-colic ligament has been divided.

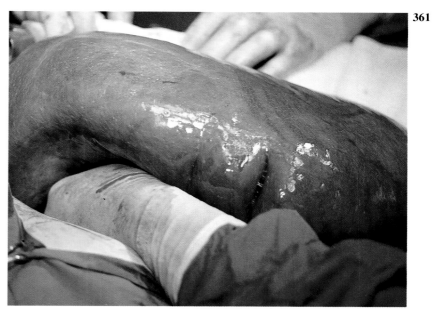

**361** The peritoneal attachments of the spleen have been divided.

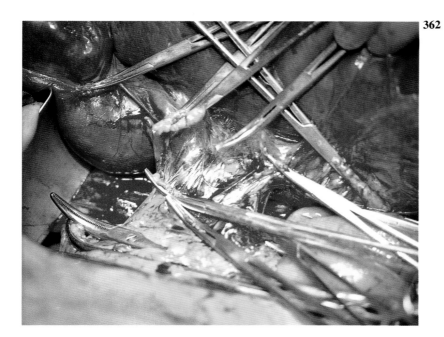

**362** The short gastric vessels have been clamped and divided – the main splenic vessels remain.

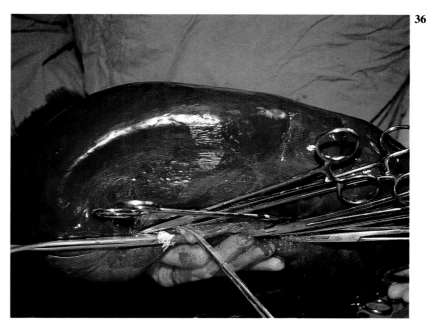

**363** The spleen has been removed and all vessels clamped.

# Kidney

Swelling arising in the loin. The lower pole can often be ballotted in a similar way to the spleen, but unless huge and reaching the anterior abdominal wall, an enlarged kidney is typically resonant to percussion due to overlying gas contained in the ascending colon on the right and descending colon on the left. It moves with respiration and unless the kidney is malpositioned, the palpating hand cannot get above the upper pole (**364-366**).

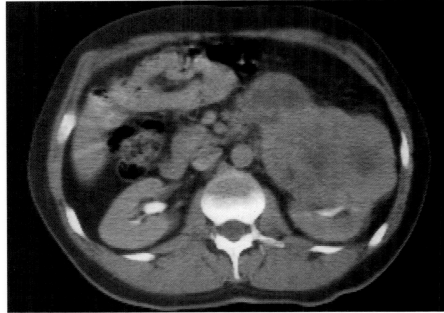

**364**

**364**   Patient with huge tumour of the left kidney, extending medially into the left renal vein but not as far as the cava.

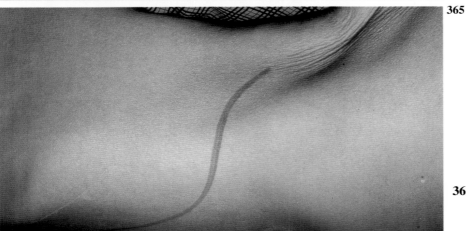

**365**

**365**   Approach to a right kidney through a curved loin incision.

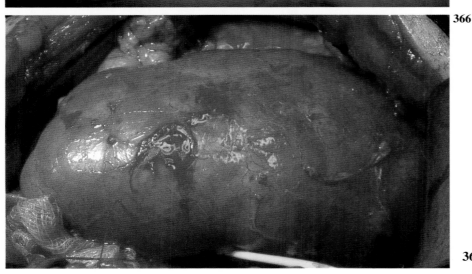

**366**

**366**   The right kidney mobilized.

# Stomach

Palpable as a boggy epigastric mass if distended. Resonant to percussion. Moves a little with respiration. A gastric carcinoma may present as a hard fixed epigastric mass. In pyloric stenosis fluid in the stomach may be detected by shaking the patient and hearing the succussion splash (**367**).

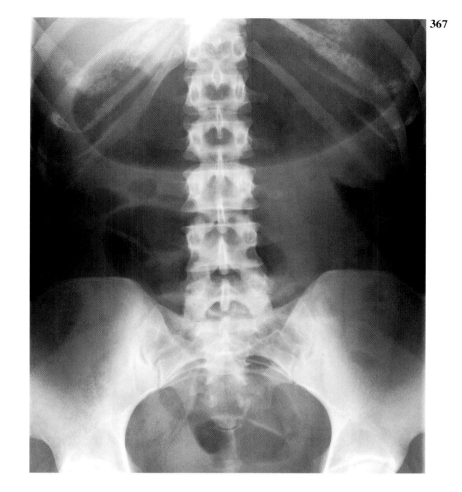

**367** A patient with acute post-operative gastric dilatation, in danger of aspiration of gastric contents into the lungs.

# Transverse Colon

Similar signs to that of an enlarged stomach but lies a little lower in the epigastrium and umbilical region.

# Sigmoid Colon

A sausage shaped and laterally mobile swelling in the left iliac fossa.

# Caecum

A squelchy resonant spherical swelling in the right iliac fossa. It can be huge and hyper-resonant in distal colonic obstruction if the ileo-caecal valve is competent (**368**).

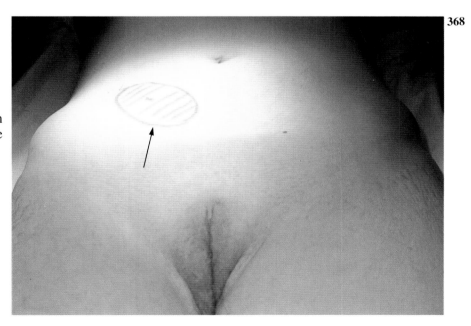

**368** A patient with a mass in the right iliac fossa (arrow) due to carcinoma of the caecum.

# Pancreas

This can seldom be palpated because of its retroperitoneal position. However, a pancreatic pseudocyst in the lesser sac may present as a dull fixed epigastric mass (**369, 370**).

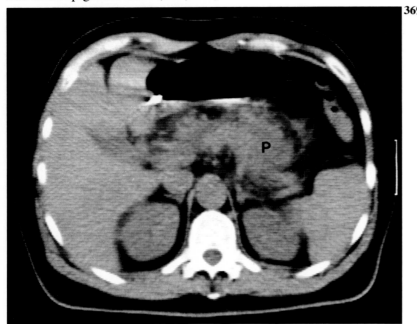

**369** CT image of a case of acute pancreatitis with a swollen, poorly defined pancreas (P) and oedema of the surrounding structures.

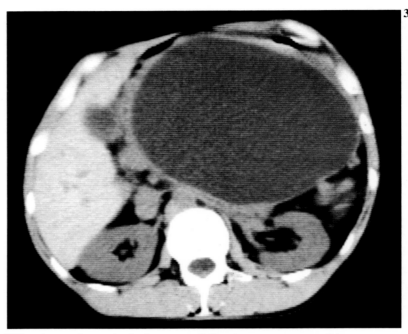

**370** A pseudocyst in the lesser sac following acute pancreatitis.

# Adrenal Glands

May mimic renal swellings and push the kidney down and on the right side the liver up, making these organs palpable, although they are not themselves diseased (**371-380**)

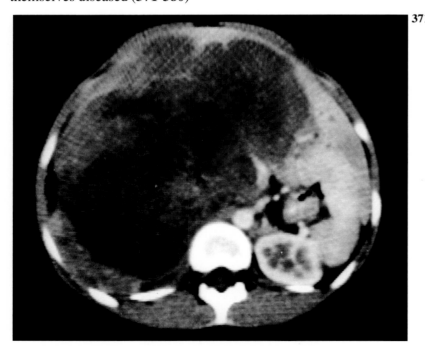

**371** A huge carcinoma of the right adrenal which involved the right lobe of the liver.

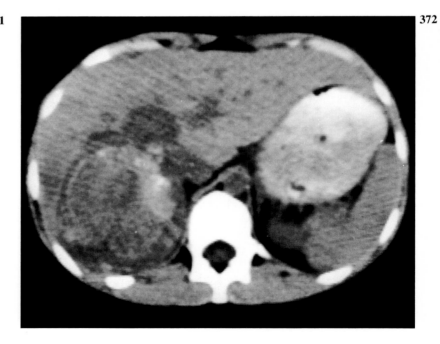

**372** This mass became smaller after treatment with chemotherapy.

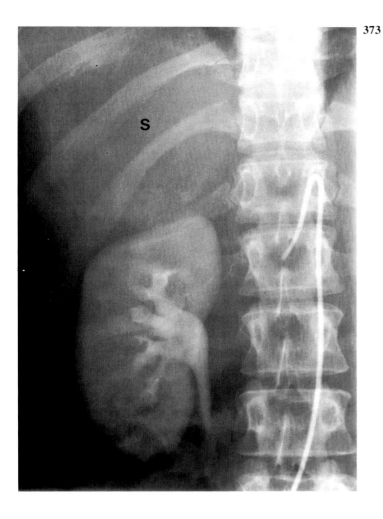

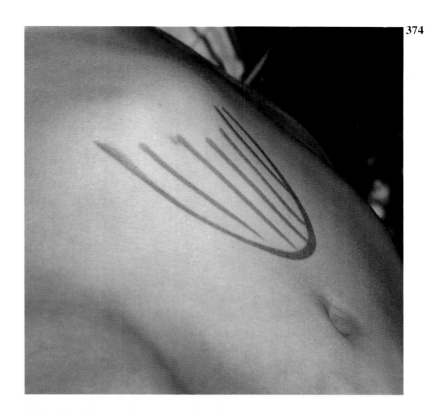

**374** Palpable swelling extending from beneath the costal margin mostly on the right side.

**373** This patient was operated on when the swelling (S) was the size indicated in his arteriogram. Note the downward displacement of the kidney.

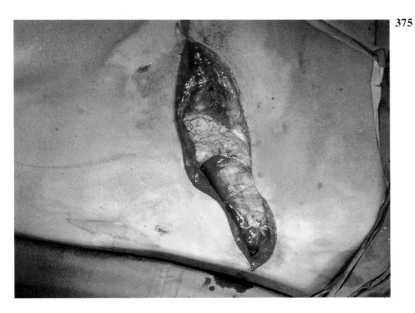

**375** Right subcostal incision.

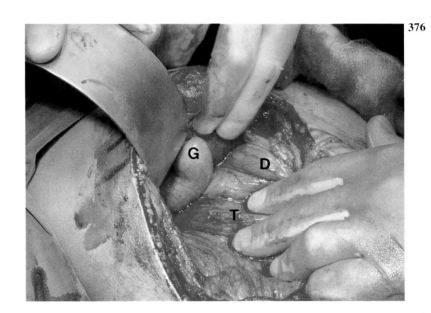

**376** The tumour (T) can be felt behind the peritoneum. Gall bladder (G); Duodenum (D).

135

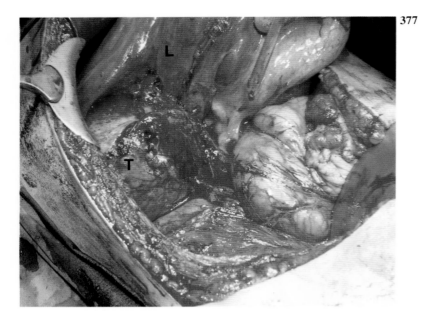

**377** The right lobe of the liver (L) dissected off the tumour (T) and lifted anteriorly.

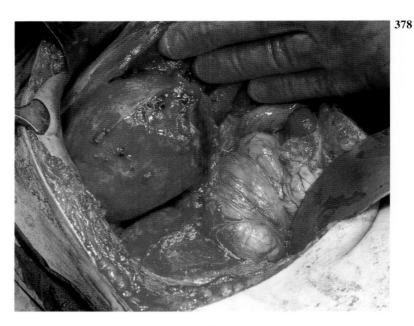

**378** The spherical tumour now mobilized.

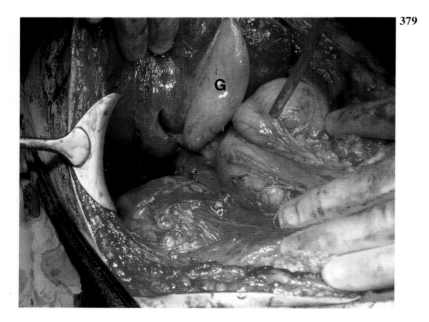

**379** The space after removal of the tumour. Gall bladder (G).

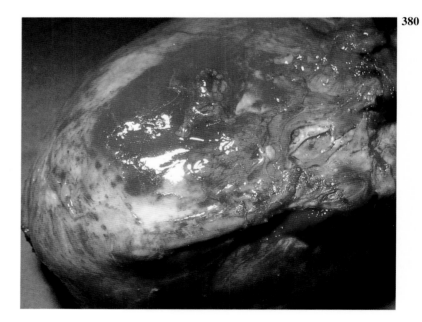

**380** The excised adrenal tumour.

# Aorta

A pulsatile swelling in the epigastric and umbilical regions, centred just to the left of the midline, usually resonant to percussion (**381**) due to overlying bowel. A large aneurysm may push the bowel aside and impinge on the anterior abdominal wall, giving a dull note to percussion which should be very gentle!

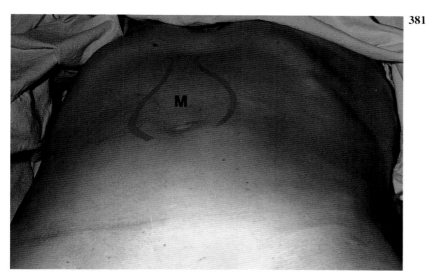

**381**    A pulsatile mass (M) in the epigastrium in a patient with an aortic aneurysm.

# Bladder

Dome shaped, swelling arising from the pelvis, dull to percussion and can reach to above the umbilicus. One can get above it (**383-384**) but not below it.

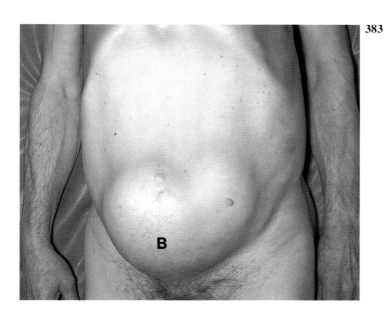

**383**    A patient with chronic retention of urine showing the large swelling suprapubically which was dull to percussion due to the enlarged bladder (B).

# Small Bowel

May be palpable in a thin person with intestinal obstruction. Visible and palpable peristalsis may be elicited in the mid abdomen, where there will be an ill-defined central swelling (**382**).

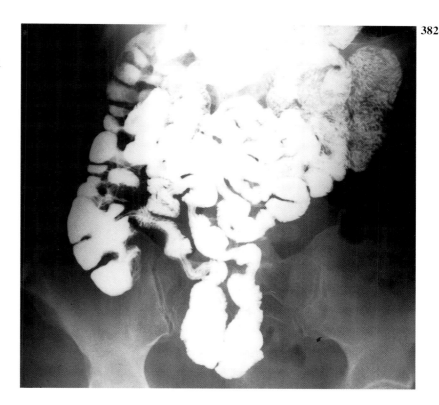

**382**    A barium follow-through showing the normal distribution of the small intestine.

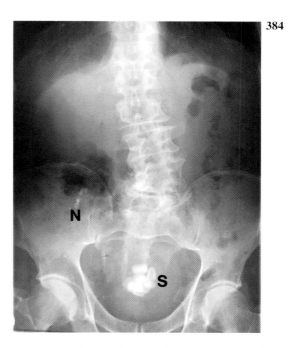

**384**    A patient with multiple large stones in the bladder (S) and also calcified lymph nodes in the right iliac fossa (N).

# Ovary

If palpable in the abdomen, is usually malignant or contains a cyst. The swelling may fill the abdominal cavity and be dull to percussion (**385-393**). Its origin in the pelvis may not be easily determined even on rectal or vaginal bimanual examination due to its mobility, but the palpating hand can reach above it. A pedunculated uterine fibroid may mimic an enlarged ovary.

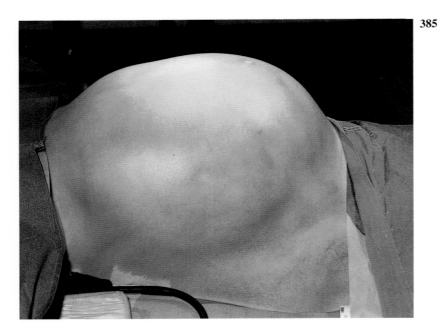

**385**    A patient with a huge ovarian cyst.

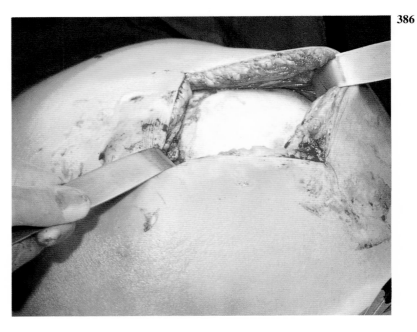

**386**    Operation on the cyst. The abdomen has been opened and the cyst is displayed.

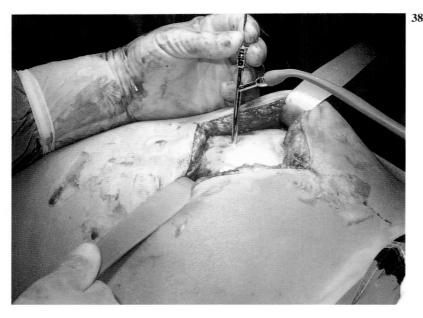

**387**    Drainage of the cyst through an aspirating needle.

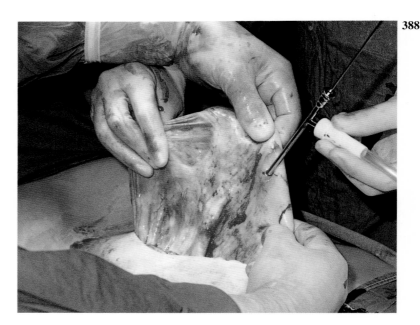

**388**    Removal of the cyst wall.

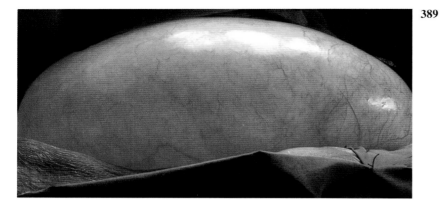

**389** An ovarian cyst transilluminated before removal, demonstrating its content of clear fluid.

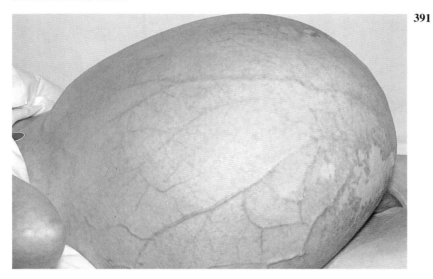

**391** A patient with a huge ovarian cyst weighing 54 lb when removed intact.

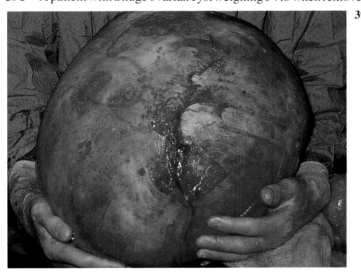

**392** The cyst removed.

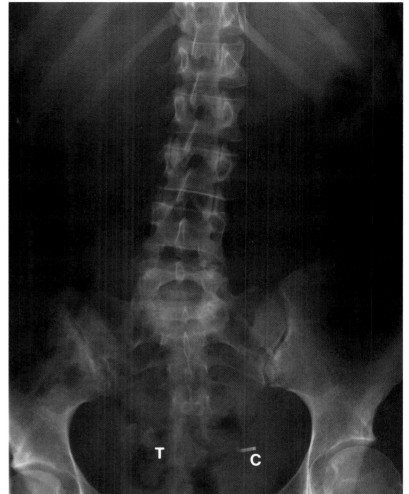

**390** X-ray of a patient with a dermoid cyst of the ovary. Teeth (T) can be seen below the right sacroiliac joint. There is an intra-uterine contraceptive device (C).

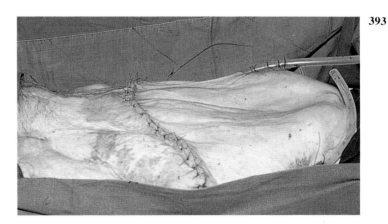

**393** The patient's abdomen after the operation.

# Uterus

Midline lower abdominal swelling, which one can get above, arises from the pelvis and is mobile. The pregnant uterus will fill the abdominal cavity and then settle a little just before delivery when the foetal head engages in the pelvis.

# 6 Some Common Surgical Conditions with Important Anatomical Features

## Obstruction of the Gastro-Intestinal Tract

**Oesophagus.** Obstruction of the gastro-oesophageal junction causes difficulty in swallowing and a sense of discomfort behind the xiphisternum. Carcinoma, stricture following gastric reflux with a hiatus hernia and achalasia are the main causes (**394-396**). The latter is a chronic disorder of oesophageal muscular co-ordination, which leads to gross dilatation of the thoracic oesophagus and overspill of food and drink into the trachea, causing a pneumonitis.

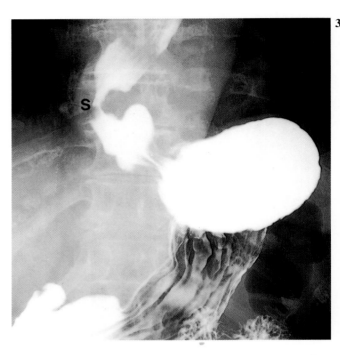

**395** Peptic stricture (S) of the oesophagus due to reflux associated with an hiatus hernia.

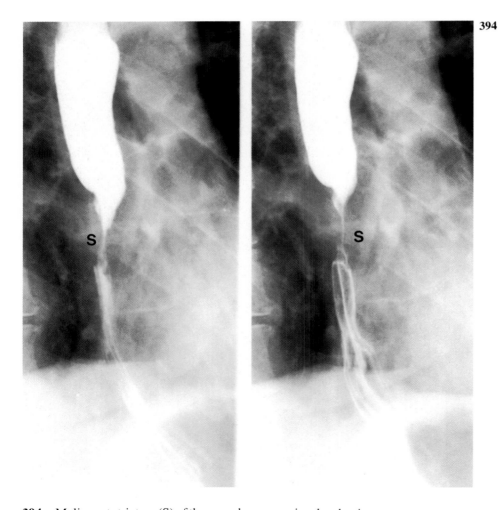

**394** Malignant stricture (S) of the oesophagus causing dysphagia.

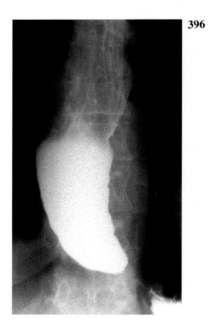

**396** Grossly dilated oesophagus due to achalasia – failure of the muscle wall of the oesophagus and the intrinsic sphincter to relax.

**Stomach.** Pyloric stenosis may present in infancy with projectile vomiting and a palpable swelling of the hypertrophied pyloric muscle (**397**). In adults, pyloric obstruction is usually secondary to a gastric cancer or chronic duodenal ulceration with fibrotic narrowing of the first part of the duodenum (**398**). Following laparotomy, paralysis of gastric muscle and paralytic ileus of the small bowel can lead to acute gastric dilatation. Malignant or fibrotic obstruction can present with vomiting of old stale food with no bile in the vomitus. There may be epigastric colicky pain and swelling with visible peristalsis passing along the stomach from the upper left hypochondrium, across to the right lower epigastrium or umbilical region. If the patient is shaken by the pelvis or thoracic cage, a succussion splash may be heard caused by the fluid and gaseous residue. Acute gastric dilatation is an insidious and potentially lethal condition that should not occur if the stomach is drained with a nasogastric tube. Some 4 to 5 days after operation, the patient, who may or may not have complained of epigastric discomfort and swelling, suddenly without warning, vomits copiously and if he is still incapacitated after surgery, he may be too weak to avoid drowning in his vomit (**399**).

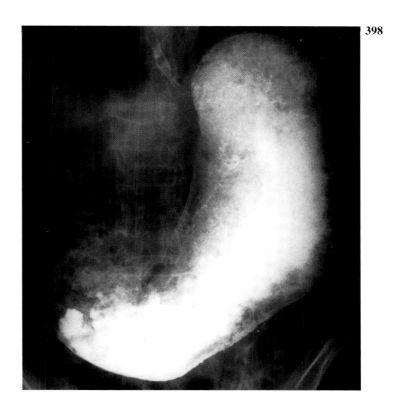

**398** Huge dilated stomach in a patient with pyloric stenosis due to fibrosis following chronic duodenal ulceration.

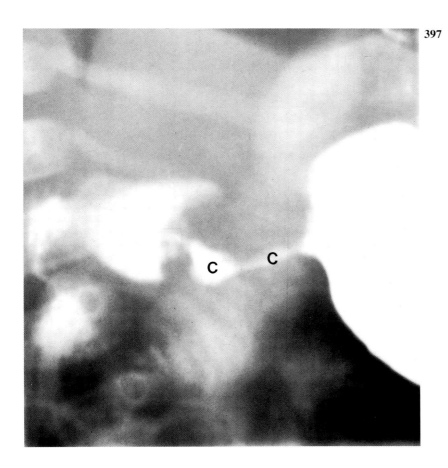

**397** Hypertrophic pyloric stenosis in an infant. The pyloric canal (c) is extremely narrow and elongated due to the hypertrophied muscle; the stomach (proximally) is dilated.

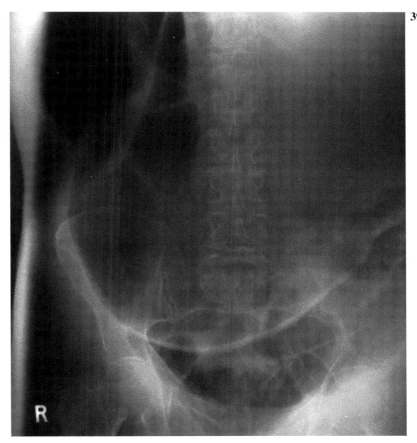

**399** Enormous post-operative gastric dilatation with the stomach extending almost into the pelvis. This patient is in great danger of dying from pneumonia due to aspiration of gastric contents.

**The Small Bowel.** Blockage of the small bowel is a common surgical emergency and is most often due to a groin hernia, intra-abdominal adhesions or Crohn's* disease. The patient complains of colicky pain centred around the umbilicus (T10) and vomiting. If unrelieved the vomitus will be faeculant in appearance and smell due to putrefaction caused by stasis. This is not true faecal vomiting, which is a rare complication of a gastro-colic fistula.

There will be central abdominal tenderness and swelling will depend on the level of obstruction. The more distal the obstruction the greater the distension. Bowel sounds are increased. Although the patient's bowels may initially function, after a few hours there is no passage of faeces or flatus. X-ray of the abdomen will show dilated loops of small bowel mostly in the centre of the abdomen, sometimes with a ladder pattern and the circumferential plicae are often visible (**400**). An X-ray taken with the patient standing erect will show fluid levels and gas overlying static pools of liquid intestinal contents (**401, 402**).

When the abdomen is inspected attention is paid to scars of previous surgery. A small right iliac fossa appendicectomy incision may, with one single band adhesion, cause intestinal obstruction 20 or more years later. The patient may point to a painful groin hernia, but in old or fat people a small obstructed hernia may be missed unless looked for specifically.

Especially notorious in being overlooked is a femoral hernia. If the hernia reduces without force, early obstruction may be relieved but repeated attempts at hernial reduction can be dangerous (see below). There may be a history of Crohn's disease or this may be the first presentation. Typically the distended ileum can be felt like a mobile sausage in the right iliac fossa (**403**). Management depends on the cause, but in all causes the stomach must be decompressed with a

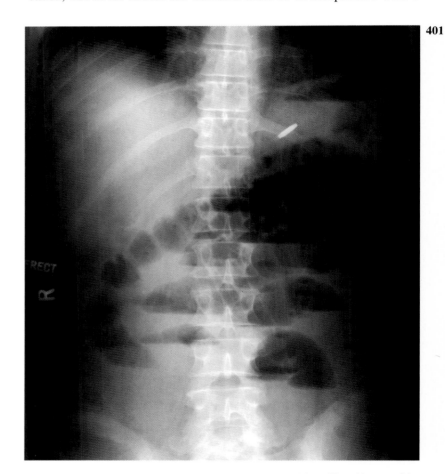

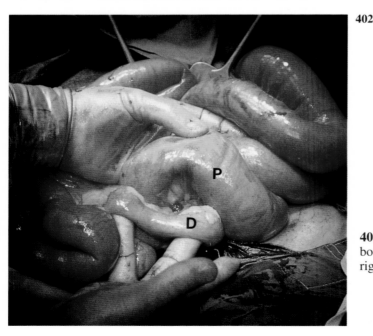

**400, 401**  Small bowel obstruction. In the supine position dilated loops of the small bowel can be seen with the valvulae conniventes going completely across the bowel lumen. In the erect X-ray in **401** multiple fluid levels can be seen arranged in a ladder pattern.

**402**  Operation for an internal hernia through the foramen of Winslow. A loop of small bowel is trapped in the foramen. Bowel proximal (P) is dilated and distal (D) in the surgeon's right hand is collapsed.

*Crohn, Burrill Bernard (1884-1983) Physician, Mount Sinai Hospital – New York.

naso-gastric tube and the fluid and electrolyte balance restored by appropriate intravenous administration. Obstructions due to adhesions may respond to these conservative measures, but most cases require surgical relief and sooner rather than later due to the danger of *strangulation*. In this process, typically seen at the neck of a hernial sac, the bowel becomes wedged in the orifice. The venous return is blocked, causing engorgement and oedema, which eventually obstructs the arterial supply resulting in death of the bowel – an extremely dangerous condition leading to generalized peritonitis. Forceful reduction of a strangulated hernia may precipitate peritonitis particularly in the femoral hernia of Richter, where only a portion of the bowel wall is strangulated, without the preceding features of intestinal obstruction.

**Large Bowel Obstruction.** This is usually due to colonic carcinoma, especially of the sigmoid, diverticular disease or volvulus. Colicky pain is suprapubic T12-L1 and may be so severe that the patient vomits. This is *not* faecal *nor* faeculant vomiting, but emptying of the gastric contents due to *pain*. Early symptoms are complete constipation for faeces and flatus and abdominal distension. A tympanitic percussion note is elicited especially in cases of volvulus or caecal distension with a competent ileocaecal valve (20%). Both these conditions are dangerous emergencies, since the caecum may burst and a twisted sigmoid may become infarcted. Abdominal X-rays will show dilated large bowel (**404-408**).

Differentiation of small and large bowel obstruction is usually straightforward (see table, page 145).

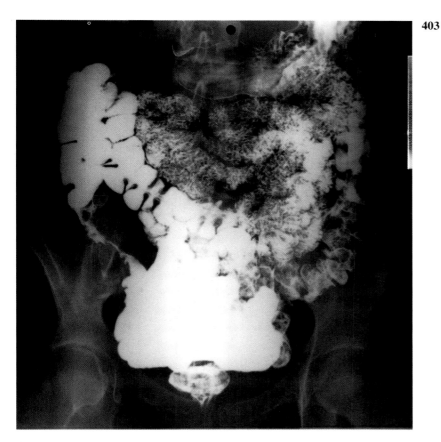

**403**  Barium follow-through study of small bowel showing narrowing of terminal ileum due to Crohn's disease.

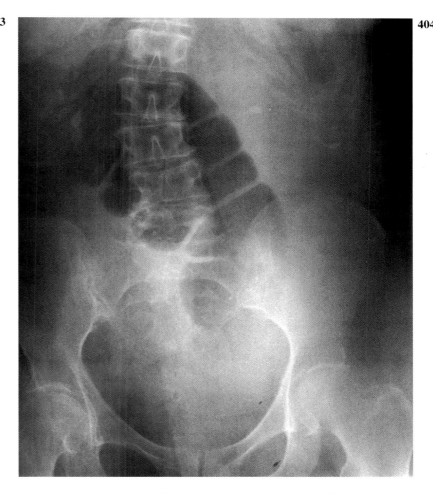

**404**  A case of volvulus of the caecum showing a grossly dilated caecum, somewhat resembling a coffee bean.

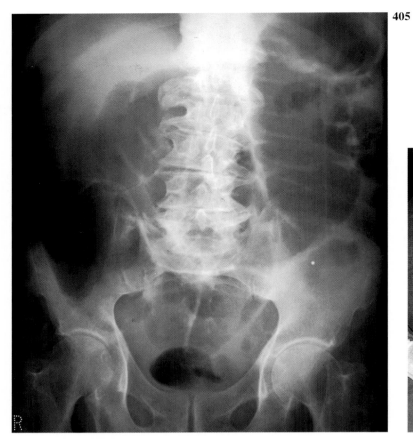

**405**

A volvulus may be managed by passing a sigmoidoscope past the point of twisting into the dilated loops. A gentle enema may give temporary relief in partial large bowel obstruction, but surgery is generally needed to decompress the bowel. If the caecum is distended surgery should be performed immediately. The large bowel can become strangulated in a hernia, although this is unusual. (**409-412**).

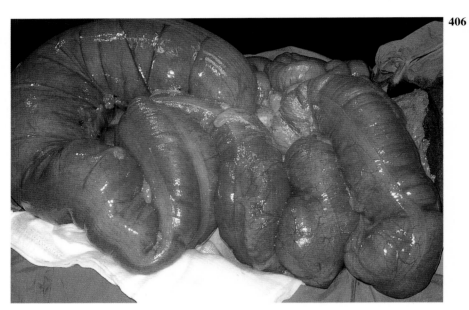

**406**

**405** Volvulus of the sigmoid colon. The huge distended sigmoid colon can be seen filling the abdomen and causing dilatation of more proximal large bowel.

**406** At operation the huge dilated loops of sigmoid colon.

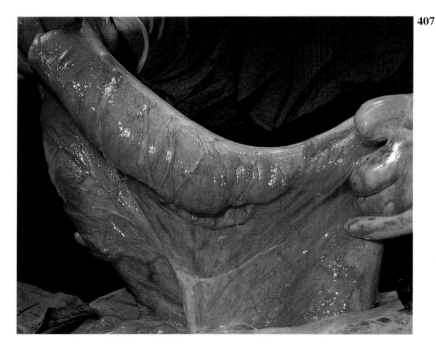

**407**

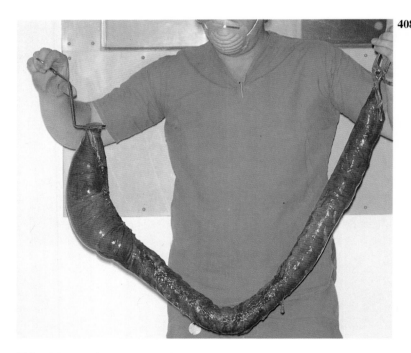

**408**

**407** The specimen mobilized.

**408** The specimen removed.

|  | SMALL BOWEL | LARGE BOWEL |
| --- | --- | --- |
| **Pain** | Central abdominal colic | Lower abdominal colic |
| **Vomiting** | **Severe**, early, becomes faeculent. Causes dehydration | Reflex associated with colic |
| **Constipation** | May not be complete until late | Complete constipation for faeces and flatus an early feature |
| **Bowel sounds** | High pitched and tinkling early | May be normal early and obstructive only later |
| **Distension** | The higher the site of obstruction, the less distension | Severe |
| **Common Causes** | Adhesions, hernia | Carcinoma of sigmoid, volvulus |
| **Straight X-ray erect and supine** | Distended small bowel in central ladder pattern. Circular folds completely across the bowel transversely. Fluid levels | Distended large bowel around periphery. Haustrations only partially crossing the bowel. Fluid levels. Distended caecum a danger sign of closed obstruction with competent ileo-caecal valve |

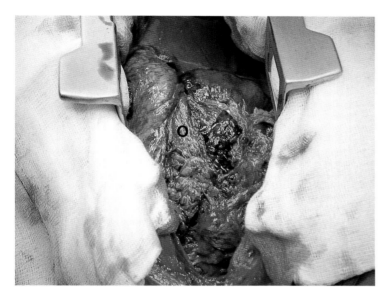

**409**   An unusual case – a strangulation of the splenic flexure of colon in a traumatic hernia of the diaphragm following a knife injury two years previously. The lesion was approached through the chest and was found to be infarcted omentum (O) overlying infarcted colon.

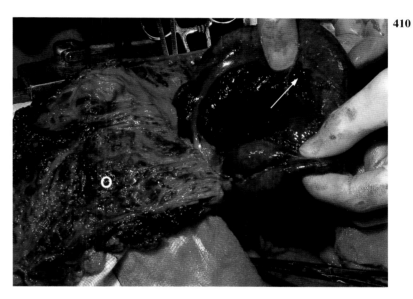

**410**   The bowel (arrow) was infarcted and removed and resection of the colon was performed in the chest. The infarcted omentum (O) can be seen on the left.

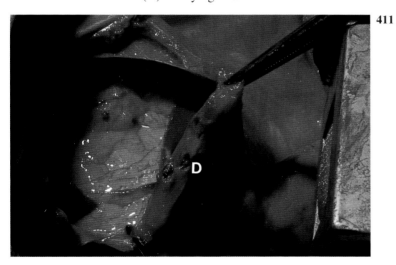

**411**   Defect in the diaphragm (D) after returning the anastomosed healthy colon to the abdomen.

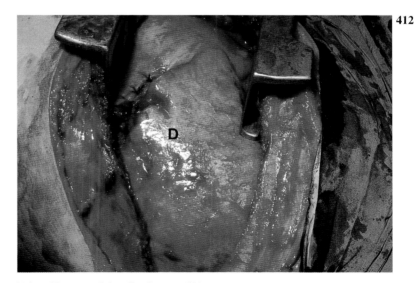

**412**   Closure of the diaphragm (D).

**Acute Appendicitis.** Typically the lumen becomes obstructed due to inflammatory oedema often associated with an intraluminal faecal concretion – a faecolith – sometimes calcified and visible on X-ray (**413**). The patient, often a child or young adult, complains of colicky central periumbilical *pain* (T10) *followed by vomiting* . This sequence is a useful pointer, since most mild infective gastro-intestinal upsets start with vomiting (the gastric inflammation) and this is followed by mid and later lower abdominal colicky pain.

In appendicitis after some hours, the pain usually settles in the right iliac fossa due to inflammatory involvement of the parietal peritoneum T12-L1. There is reflex spasm of the muscles of the anterior abdominal wall overlying the appendix. Palpation in this region will aggravate the pain and abdominal muscle spasm. As the abdomen is pressed the abdominal wall becomes increasingly rigid –*guarding*. There may be a low grade pyrexia, neutrophil leucocytosis, and the patient is disinterested in food and has a furred tongue and foetor. A

patient who can tuck into a steak and chips is almost certainly *not* suffering from acute appendicitis, especially if the external iliac artery can be palpated on the right side. Since the appendix is mobile and can lie in different places there may be special signs and symptoms because of the abdominal relations (**414-417**).

A retrocaecal inflamed appendix lying on the psoas muscle may cause flexion and internal rotation of the hip due to psoas spasm. If the leg is extended passively this will cause pain in the right iliac fossa. An appendix lying in the pelvis may irritate the rectum causing diarrhoea and on rectal examination there will be tenderness in the right side of the pelvis. An acutely inflamed appendix, lying on the obturator internus muscle posteriorly and deep in the pelvis, will cause pain if the flexed hip is internally rotated.

An anterior lying inflamed appendix may irritate the parietal peritoneum overlying the gall bladder and mimic disease of that organ. If not removed, an inflamed appendix may rupture and cause

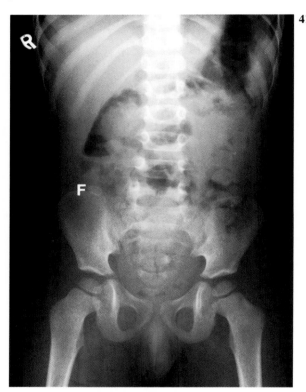

**413**

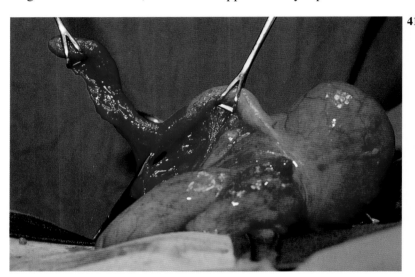

**414**

**414–416** Examples of acute appendicitis. In each case the organ is oedematous and red in colour. In **416** there is a perforation in the base. A small yellow spot can be seen where pus is being extruded.

**413** Straight X-ray of a child with appendicitis. A large faecolith (F) can be seen just above the pelvis on the right side.

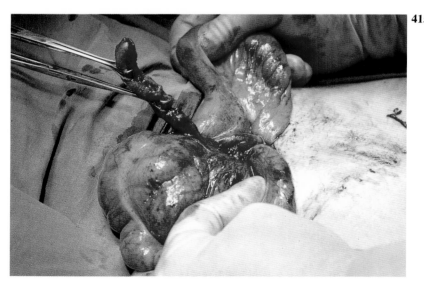

**415**

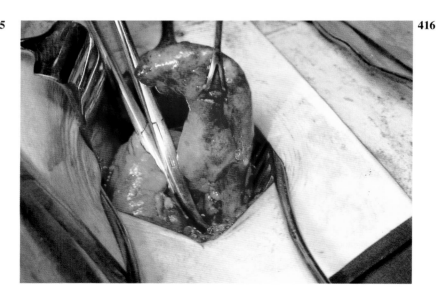

**416**

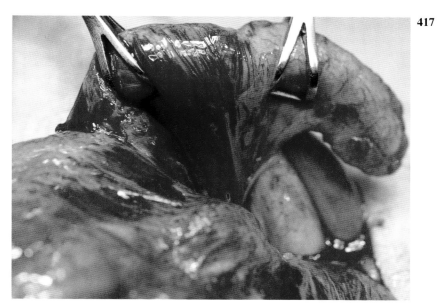

**417** High power view of acute appendicitis.

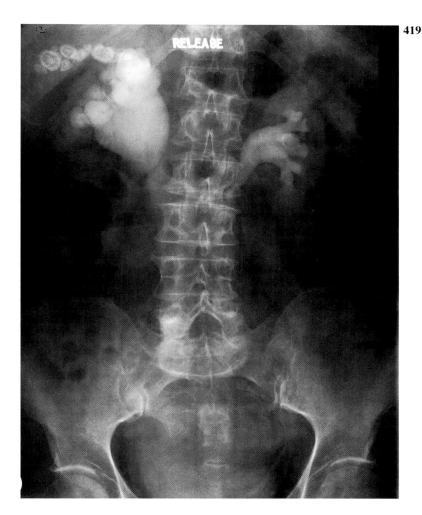

**419** A complicated case with bilateral hydronephrosis due to inflammatory changes around an aortic aneurysm. Multiple radio-opaque gall stones are also shown. Only approximately 10% of cases of gallstones are radio-opaque. The ring appearance indicates different stages in the gall stone formation when the calcium content of the bile was high.

**417** generalized peritonitis or it may form a localized abscess with a surrounding mass of fibrinous adhesions to bowel and body wall (**418**). Such a phlegmon or appendix mass will usually resolve spontaneously with conservative management. An abscess in the pelvis may discharge pus into the rectum.

**Cholecystitis.** Inflammation of the gall bladder is usually associated with gall stones (**419, 420**). An acute attack presents with epigastric

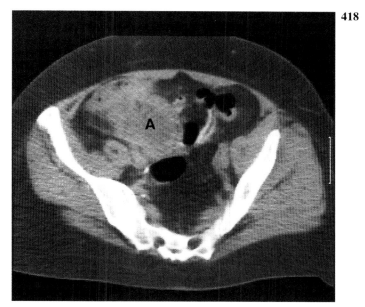

**418** An appendix mass. Abscess (A) is contained by adhesions.

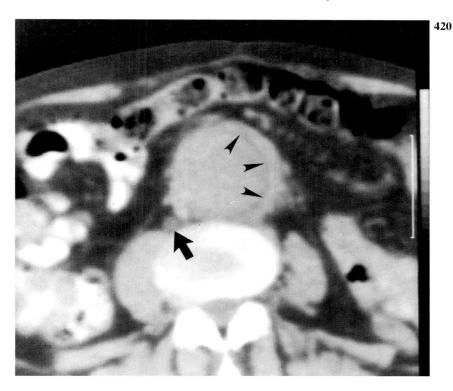

**420** CT of same case as **419** showing the aneurysm and dilated right ureter (arrow). The periaortic inflammation (arrowheads) has already obstructed the left ureter (reproduced with permission of *Clinical Radiology*).

pain T8, 9, vomiting and indigestion. It is usually precipitated by fatty food, which stimulates contraction of the gall bladder by causing release of the hormone cholecystokinin from the duodenal wall. Pain may localize to the right subcostal region if the parietal peritoneum (also T8, 9) is involved in the inflammation. With the surgeon's hand placed under the costal margin, downward movement of the gall bladder when a breath is taken causes pain and the patient stops the intake of breath with a gasp, Murphy's* sign. The posterior parietal peritoneum may be irritated causing pain in the back of the chest on the right side and hyperaesthesia of the skin (Boas'† sign).

**Pancreatitis.** An inflamed retroperitoneal pancreas causes pain in the back over L1, 2 spines. As pancreatic enzymes become liberated into the peritoneal cavity there will be generalized abdominal pain, vomiting, rigid abdominal muscles and absent bowel sounds due to peritonitis. The serum amylase level will usually be raised above 1000 international units. Severe haemorrhagic pancreatitis with auto-digestion of the pancreas may cause blockage of the common bile duct with jaundice, renal failure and pseudocyst formation in the lesser sac. There may be erosion of the superior mesenteric artery or its middle colic branch, with necrosis of the transverse colon and intra-abdominal haemorrhage.

**Acute Peritonitis.** The peritoneum will become irritated and inflamed if its normal bland peritoneal fluid environment is changed to any noxious material. Blood from a ruptured viscus, urine, bile, pancreatic juice and intestinal contents will all cause peritonitis. The clinical features are generalized abdominal pain, rigidity of the abdominal muscles, paralysis of intestinal motility. Often there will be free gas in the abdomen if the intestine is perforated and this can be seen on erect chest X-ray as gas under the diaphragm (**421**).

In upper abdominal peritonitis the diaphragm will be irritated, causing pain referred over one or both shoulders (C3, 4 and 5 phrenic) and shallow respiration.

**Perforated Duodenal Ulcer.** Perforated duodenal ulcer usually occurs through an acute anterior duodenal ulcer (**422**) but there may be a history of chronic ulceration with hunger pains relieved by food (**423**). The patient can state the exact moment and usually remembers vividly what he was doing when the pain, like a deep stab in the upper abdomen, occurred. The pain causes the patient to remain still because all movements increase the agony. The abdominal wall feels like a rigid board. There will be no bowel sounds. The pain is often referred from the diaphragm to the right shoulder.

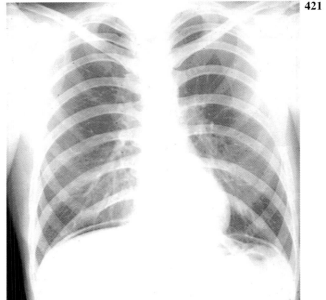

**421**  Patient with a perforated duodenal ulcer showing air under both domes of the diaphragm.

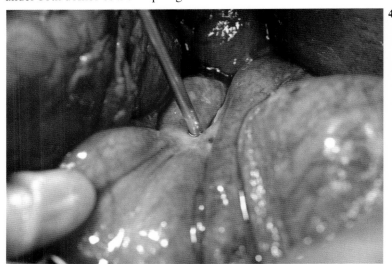

**422**  Operation on a patient with a perforated duodenal ulcer. The probe is inserted into the perforation through the front of a chronic duodenal ulcer.

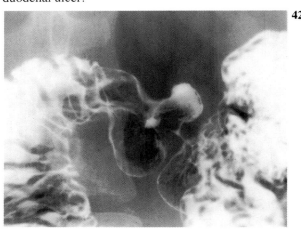

**423**  Barium meal showing scarred duodenal cap with a central ulcer crater and cloverleaf trefoil deformity.

*Murphy, John Benjamin (1857-1916) Surgeon – Chicago.
†Boas, Ismar Isidor (1858-1938) Physician – Berlin.

148

**Perforated Diverticulum.** Colonic diverticula are common and often symptomless (**424, 425**). An inflamed diverticulum may perforate or bleed. As with a perforated duodenal ulcer the onset of symptoms from a ruptured diverticulum is usually sudden, although there may be a history of lower abdominal pain due to previous attacks of diverticulitis with localized left iliac fossa pain. In this case a pericolic abscess may have perforated into the general peritoneal cavity. Pus is bad enough, but the escape of faeces into the peritoneal cavity causes a high mortality, even when recognized quickly and operated on before the patient lapses into a shocked septicaemic state. As with a duodenal perforation, there will be board-like rigidity and absent bowel sounds. Tachycardia and hypotension may occur early.

In some cases the differential diagnosis between a perforated duodenal ulcer and a perforated diverticulum can be difficult, especially if the patient has been on long-term corticosteroid treatment, which masks the symptoms and signs and therefore the gravity of both conditions.

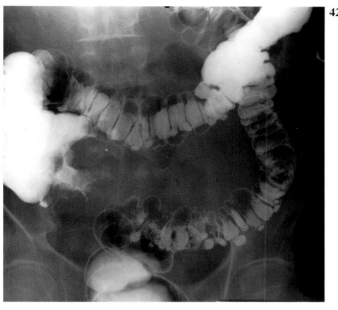

**424**

**424** Barium enema on a patient with multiple diverticula, especially in the sigmoid colon. The caecum is deformed by a carcinoma.

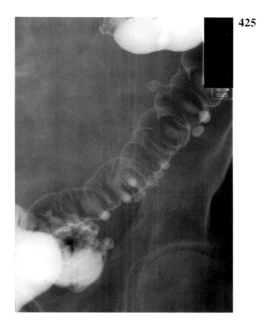

**425**

**425** Another barium enema view of diverticular disease.

**Ruptured Spleen.** There is usually a history of a blow on the left lower ribs, one or more of which may be fractured (**426, 427**). There is localized pain over the fractured ribs and guarding or rigidity under the left costal margin T9–11. There is likely to be pain over the left shoulder tip referred by the phrenic nerve due to diaphragmatic irritation, C3, 4 and 5. There will be signs of bleeding with tachycardia and hypotension. Lavage of the peritoneal cavity will reveal fresh blood.

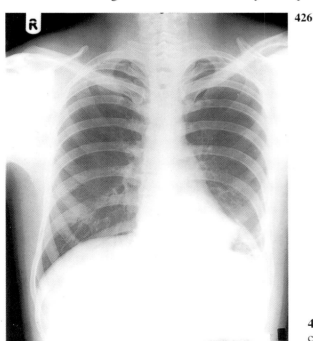

**426**

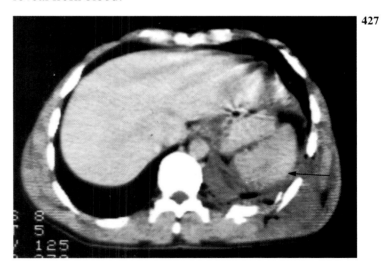

**427**

**427** CT scan showing a rupture of the spleen (arrow) which is markedly heterogeneous in a case with fractured ribs.

**426** An X-ray of a patient with fractured ribs in the left lower chest. The costophrenic angle is blunt due to an effusion. The fractures are not well shown.

**Ruptured Liver.** Identical clinical features to those of a ruptured spleen but the symptoms and signs are on the right (**428-431**).

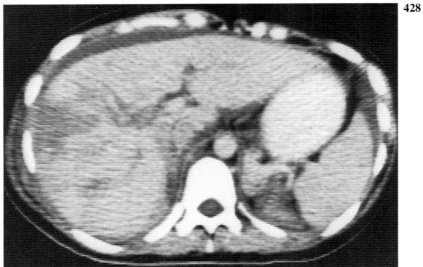

**428**

**428** Rupture of the liver following a blunt injury from a road traffic accident. The laterally placed laceration is well shown during contrast enhancement.

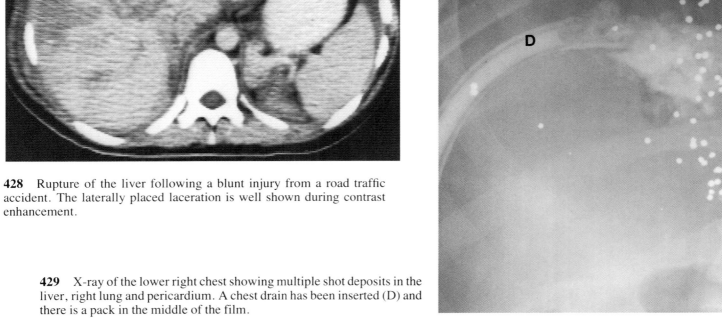

**429**

**429** X-ray of the lower right chest showing multiple shot deposits in the liver, right lung and pericardium. A chest drain has been inserted (D) and there is a pack in the middle of the film.

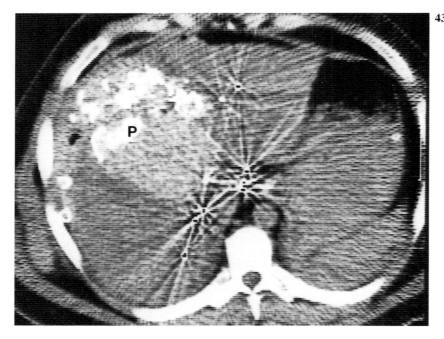

**430**

**430** Multiple shot gun pellets embedded in the liver from a burst of shot at point blank range. A pack (P) was inserted as a temporary measure at emergency surgery. There is an extensive haematoma around the pack.

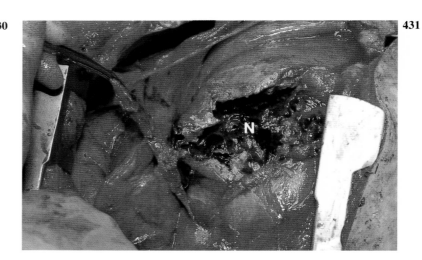

**431**

**431** The liver was approached through the right chest, the diaphragm opened, the necrotic bleeding lesion (N) can be seen in the middle of the right lobe of the liver on the diaphragmatic surface.

**Ureteric Colic.** The pain is colicky in nature, very severe and accompanied by vomiting, the pain is referred from loin to groin and testis or labia T12-L1. Between the episodes of agony there is still a residual burning pain. The cause is usually a stone that has blocked the ureter, which is desperately trying to expel the hard foreign body (**432-437**).

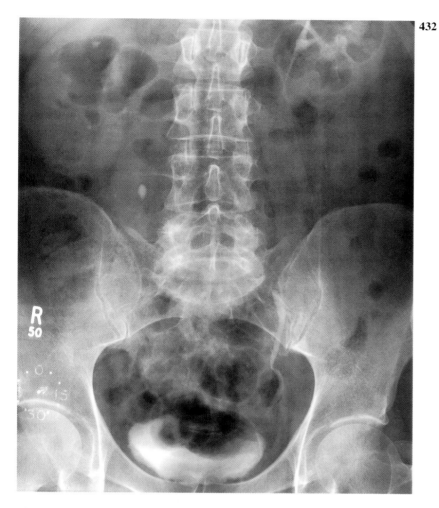

432  X-ray showing a stone in the line of the right ureter.

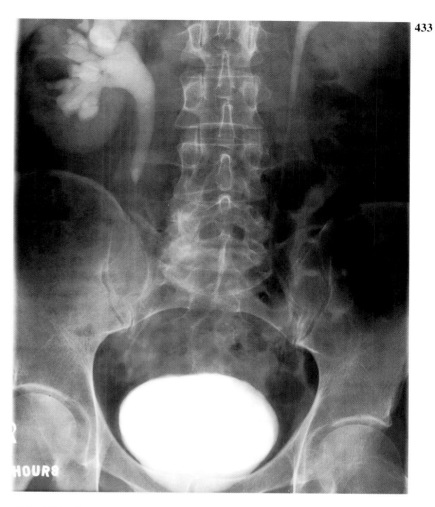

433  This diagnosis was confirmed by IVU showing blockage of the ureter at the point of the stone.

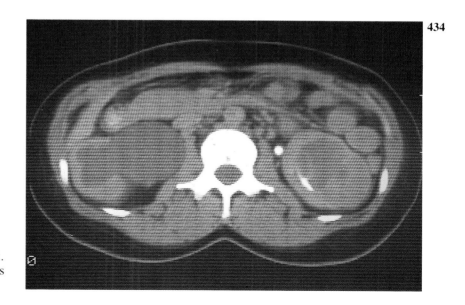

434  A CT scan showing bilateral hydronephrosis, more marked on the right. No evidence of dilated ureters. Thus pelviureteric junction obstruction was diagnosed.

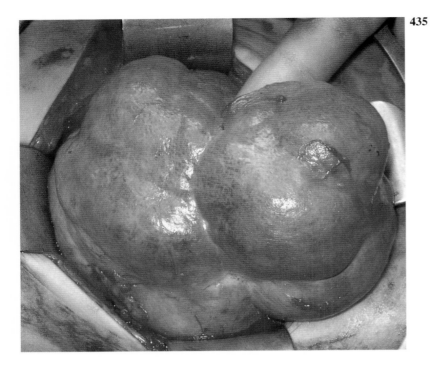

**435** Operation on hydronephrosis.

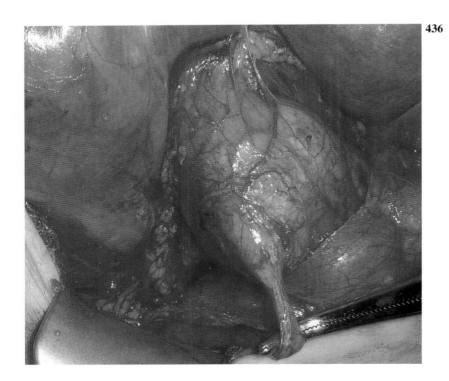

**436** The junction of dilated pelvis with ureter can be seen. The forceps demonstrate a normal ureter.

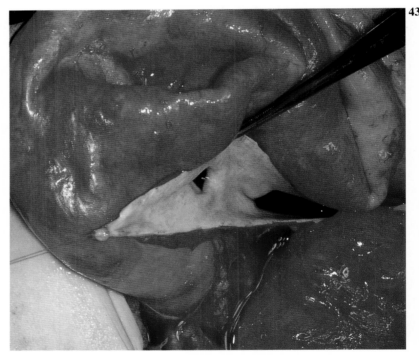

**437** The narrowing of the junction can be seen from within the lumen of the ureter.

**Ruptured Aortic Aneurysm.** The patient is usually an elderly male who may have had a history of a pulsating abdominal swelling and backache, T12, L1, 2, but the rupture can present without the lesion having been previously recognized. The rupture causes a sudden very severe central abdominal pain T10, radiating to the back. If the aneurysm has ruptured through the aortic wall into the retroperitoneal tissues without breaching the peritoneum, then there may be only moderate hypotension and tachycardia. This variety of rupture has a good prognosis if operated on immediately (**438**). If the aneurysm has ruptured freely into the peritoneal cavity, there will be severe shock and the pulsating swelling may not even have been felt. Such patients may be wrongly diagnosed as suffering from a myocardial infarction.

**Obstruction of the Renal Pelvis and Ureter.** This can result in gross proximal dilation of the upper urinary collecting system.

**Acute Retention of Urine.** The patient, usually an elderly male, with a history of a poor urinary stream and frequency, presents with severe suprapubic pain T12, L1 and is unable to pass urine. The bladder can be palpated as a dome shaped tender swelling dull to percussion above the pubis. If there has been preceding partial obstruction, the bladder may have already been stretched and can extend to above the umbilicus, still dull to percussion since it pushes the anterior parietal peritoneum away from the transversalis fascia as it enlarges.

**Ruptured Ectopic Pregnancy.** The patient, a woman of childbearing age, may have just missed a period. The tubal pregnancy ruptures and bleeds causing localized parietal peritoneal irritation in the right or left iliac fossa (T12-L1) with pain, guarding and rigidity (**439**). Pain from the ovary itself may be referred to the groin and along the adductor side of the thigh (L2, 3, 4).

Tachycardia and hypotension indicate haemorrhage and surgery should be performed as soon as the shock has been treated by rapid intravenous infusion, preferably of blood.

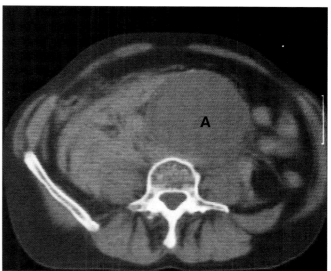

**438**

**438**  CT scan showing an 8 cm aortic aneurysm (A). The tissue planes around are distorted, especially on the right. This was due to retroperitoneal haematoma, secondary to rupture.

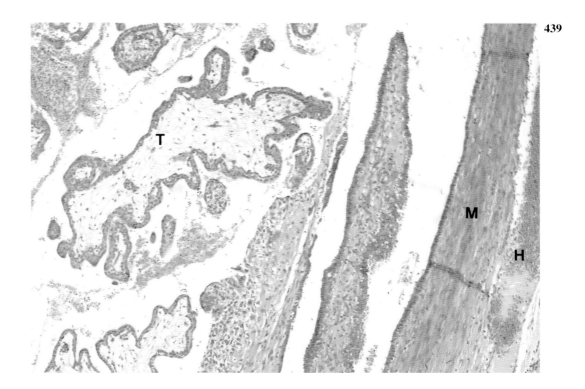

**439**

**439**  A ruptured ectopic pregnancy. The lumen of the tube contains blood and trophoblastic villi (T) and there is haemorrhage (H) into the muscle wall (M).

**Haemorrhoids.** Some degree of engorgement of the submucous veins and arteriovenous cushions in the anal canal is normal during defaecation, but if these varicosities become enlarged they will be traumatized by a hard motion and bleed – a first degree pile. Further enlargement results in the pile prolapsing as a lump and returning spontaneously with or without digital help – a second degree pile. Later, the pile fails to return even when pushed – a third degree pile (**440-443**). Although bleeding and prolapsing of anal lumps are unpleasant, piles only become painful if they are inflamed, thrombosed or acutely strangulated. This latter is an ''attack of piles'' never to be forgotten by the patient (**444**). The piles, usually at 3, 7 and 11 o'clock, with the patient lying supine in the lithotomy position, prolapse through the anus and become gripped by the anal sphincter.

The venous return is blocked, oedema occurs and the piles may swell to the size of plums. To see three such tumours arising from the anus is alarming for an inexperienced doctor and terrifying for the patient, since they are also very painful. Gentle pressure may reduce the piles if they are seen early, otherwise the patient requires sedation, cold packs to the piles and the foot of the bed raised. They will shrivel up after about a week and may spontaneously atrophy or more likely require surgical removal. Some surgeons advocate operating in the acute oedematous phase. The rectum may itself prolapse out of the anus. This usually occurs in elderly women with weakness of the levatores ani muscles. It may be accompanied by uterine prolapse (**445, 446**).

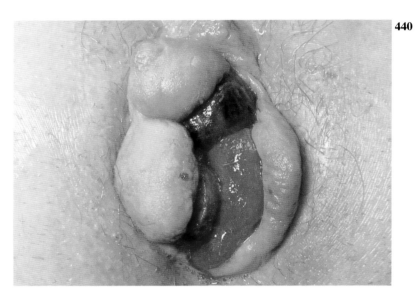

**440**  Third degree piles.

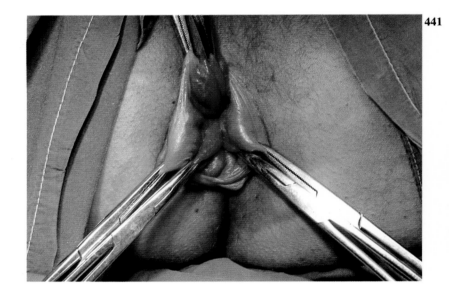

**441-443**  Operation on third degree piles.

**441**  The piles are everted and the sphincter dilated.

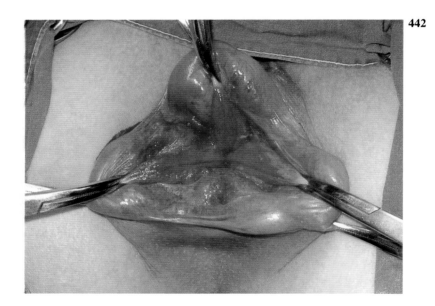

**442**  Further dilatation.

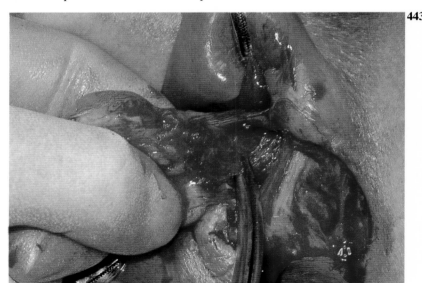

**443**  Excision with suture ligation of the base of the piles.

154

The above consideration of a few typical surgical conditions of the abdomen is given in an attempt to bring to life the purpose of studying anatomy. It is in no way a text of surgery or surgical treatment. It will be appreciated that the quicker a complaint or correct diagnosis is made or a list of probabilities constructed, the sooner treatment can begin and the greater are the chances of a speedy recovery. An understanding as well as a knowledge of anatomy is essential to correlate the patient's symptoms, signs and special investigations with the pathology.

*The dimension of time is central to all surgery.* Not only must a working diagnosis be made quickly, but the decision whether or not to operate and when, must be taken. An error may cost the patient his life and a mistake will always be revealed not only to the surgeon, but also to his medical and nursing colleagues. This is one of the fascinating attractions of surgery. Mistakes will always be recognized by an honest surgeon and hopefully lessons are learned so that they are not repeated.

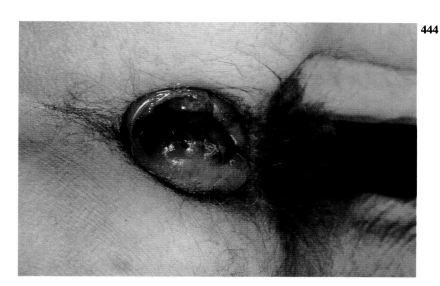

**444** Acute prolapse of strangulated piles. The piles have been gripped by the anal sphincter which has caused venous blockage, oedema and arterial occlusion. These are the features of strangulation leading to the death of the tissue that has been strangulated.

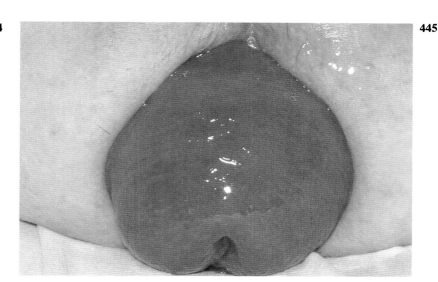

**445** Full thickness prolapse of the rectum.

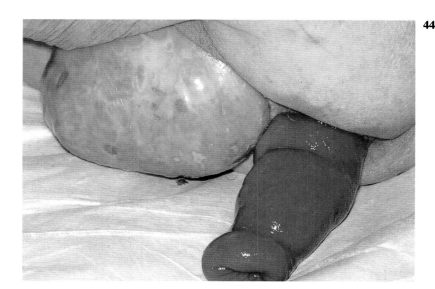

**446** Full thickness prolapse of the rectum together with complete prolapse of the uterus.

## When Not to Operate

If a patient is severely malnourished as in starvation or chronic infection following multiple operations or as a result of intestinal fistulae, healing following surgery may not take place, despite otherwise perfect surgical technique. In such cases it is in the patient's best interests to defer major procedures, such as bowel resection. Only life-saving procedures should be undertaken, for example, draining an abscess or decompressing an obstructed bowel.

The nutritional state is restored by compassionate nursing, feeding via the enteral or, if that is not possible, a parenteral route, until suddenly one day – and it often appears that way, the patient feels and looks better, develops an appetite and starts gaining weight. He is now in *"positive nitrogen balance"* and definitive surgery can be undertaken with comparative safety. It may take weeks or even months before a seriously ill patient's nutritional state is restored.

## The Surgical Importance of Blood Supply

Organs deprived of blood will die and the necrotic tissue is susceptible to infection, resulting in a moist purulent gangrene. There is a considerable safety factor of *collateral blood vessels* in most organs and this is especially so if, once again, the dimension of time is taken into account. Severe, slow atherosclerotic vascular occlusion of intestinal arteries can be well tolerated, provided at least one of the three main visceral arteries, coeliac, superior and inferior mesenteric, remains widely patent. Acute occlusion of the superior mesenteric is not tolerated. **447** shows nearly the whole small intestine which sloughed and was extruded from the surgical wound of a patient whose superior mesenteric artery suddenly occluded. Recovery took 18 months of skillful nursing (**448, 449**).

**447**

**447** Necrotic small bowel extruded from the abdominal wound in a patient whose superior mesenteric artery had been occluded.

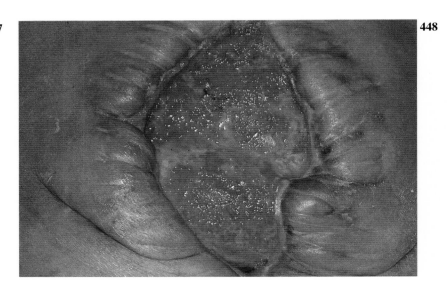
**448**

**448** The patient was in negative nitrogen balance for nearly a year. It took more than a year for the wound to heal.

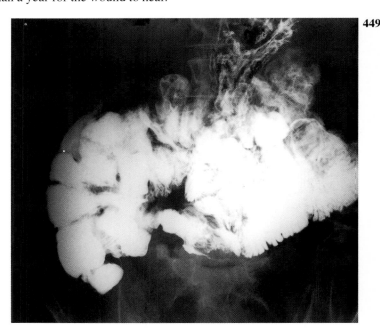
**449**

**449** Small bowel enema two years later showing some residual jejunum which is only approximately one-eighth of the normal length of the small bowel.

The remarkable collateral vascular network in the stomach has been mentioned. When bowel is resected, the chances of a perfect union of the anastomotic reconstruction depends on a number of factors:

1 Nutritional and metabolic state of the patient. If the nitrogen balance is negative healing will not take place.

2 The contents of the viscus. The stomach and upper small bowel heal well, ileum and proximal colon less well but usually satisfactorily. With distal colon and rectum, there is a risk of leakage of bacterial laden faecal contents, which may cause the anastomosis to fail. For this reason great care is taken to wash mechanically and in most centres reduce the bacterial content of the bowel with antibiotics, prior to colonic surgery.

3 The surgical technique. The opposing walls must be approximated carefully without tension. No holes must be left, but the stitches must not be pulled too tight or they will occlude the blood vessels at the edge of the anastomosis and this will lead to swelling, necrosis and leakage of bowel content. Many different techniques are advocated with a variety of materials, but the principal objective is always the same.

4 The blood supply to the cut ends (**450-453**). This is precarious in the oesophagus due to its segmental blood supply, but any piece of bowel may be rendered ischaemic if it is too extensively mobilized, if it is pulled under tension to perform the anastomosis or if the patient already has narrowing or blockage of the arteries supplying the viscus in question.

The blood supply of the spleen and kidneys are critical since sudden occlusion of the main vessels can seldom be tolerated without extensive infarction. The liver with its dual arterial and portal venous blood supply has more reserve. Occlusion of the common hepatic artery is often well tolerated, since flow in the portal vein, normally providing two-thirds of the blood supply to the liver, increases and collateral arteries rapidly open up in the peritoneal attachments of the liver. Likewise, sudden obstruction of the portal vein may not lead to severe liver parenchymatous damage, although the ensuing portal hypertension may cause ascites and bleeding from oesophageal varices. If both the artery and the vein are suddenly occluded, death will follow in a few hours, unless a new liver can be grafted as an emergency (**454-457**).

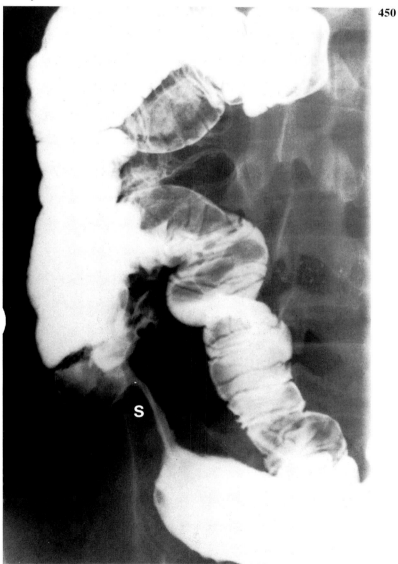

**450**

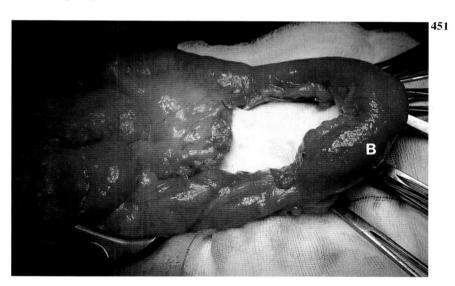

**451**

**451** The mesentery of the diseased portion of ileum has been ligated and divided. The devascularized bowel has turned a dusky brick red colour (B).

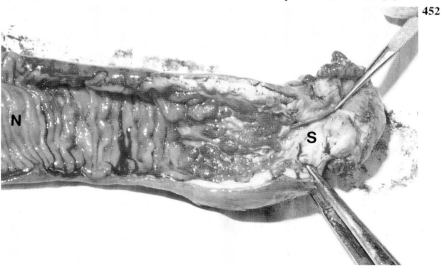

**452**

**450** Barium follow-through showing a stricture (S) of the ileum proximal to a previous anastomosis (Crohn's disease, **451-453**).

**452** The removed specimen opened. The probe demonstrates the stricture (S) with the thickened bowel wall of Crohn's disease. Normal ileal mucosa on left (N).

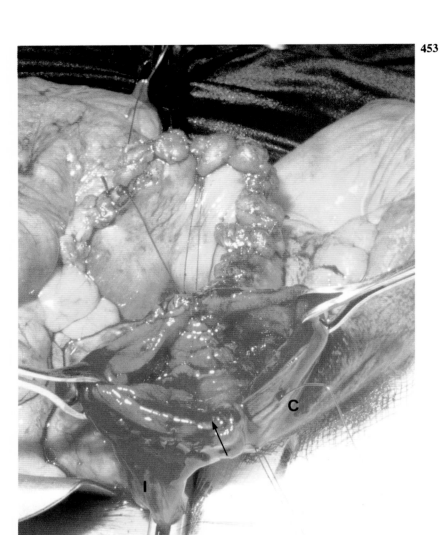

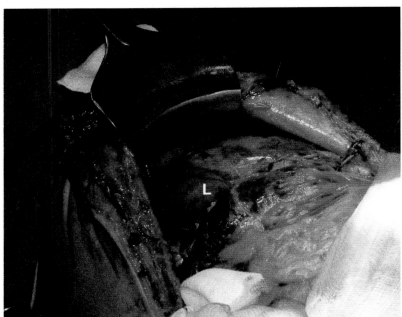

**454** Total infarction of a liver (L) transplant in which the hepatic artery and portal vein were both occluded (**455**).

**453** The ileum (I) is being anastomosed to the transverse colon (C). The posterior walls have been approximated by sutures. The edges of the anterior walls held by forceps are bleeding freely (arrow) indicating a good blood supply, a necessary requirement for healing.

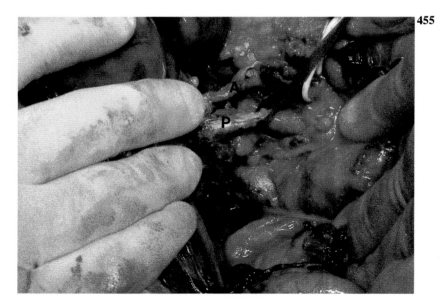

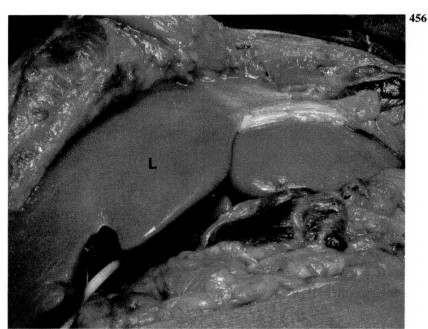

**455** There was no blood supply from either the hepatic artery (A) or portal vein (P).

**456** A new liver (L) was transplanted and satisfactorily vascularized. The patient is well 3 years later with normal liver function.

# Subhepatic Space of Rutherford Morison*

As mentioned in Chapter 1, this is the "Piccadilly Circus" for the general surgeon where many things happen and it is essential to know one's way about, within a 4-cm radius are the following structures.

1  The liver – right and caudate lobes.
2  The gall bladder.
3  Duodenum.
4  The free edge of the lesser omentum with bile duct, hepatic artery and portal vein.
5  Head of pancreas and ampulla of Vater.
6  Right renal vein.
7  Vena cava.
8  Right renal artery.
9  Right ureter.
10  Right kidney.
11  Right adrenal.

Pathology can occur in any of these structures and spread from one to another. Most common in surgical practice are acute cholecystitis and perforated duodenal ulcer.

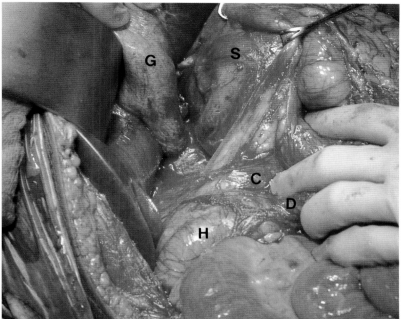

**457**  Kocher's manoeuvre. The forceps are holding the greater curve of the stomach (S) upwards and out of the wound. The gall bladder (G) is under the surgeon's hand on the left. In the sub-hepatic space can be seen the hepatic flexure of the colon (H). The surgeon's middle finger overlies the inferior vena cava (C). The mobilized duodenum (D) lies between the middle and ring fingers.

# The Anatomy of the Abdominal Aortic Aneurysm

This is surgically important both in elective aneurysm resection and as an emergency in cases of rupture. It is of historical interest that Astley Cooper (**458**) performed anatomical dissections every morning between 6 and 7.30 a.m before routine work so as to be constantly familiar with topographical anatomy. He successfully ligated an aneurysm in 1817 for the first time, before the introduction of general anaesthesia. In the crowded auditorium of the operating theatre at Guy's Hospital, this remarkable surgeon performed a laparotomy and within a few minutes turned to address the audience of students. "Gentlemen, I have the pleasure of informing you that the aorta is now hooked around my finger." The poor patient survived the procedure, but developed sepsis from which he died some days later.

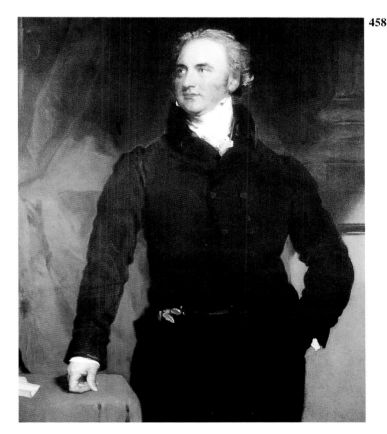

**458**  Photograph of a painting of Astley Cooper which is in the Royal College of Surgeons of England.

It is thought that the flow of blood to the kidneys – 25% of the cardiac output – determines the usual site of the commencement of abdominal aneurysms below the renal arteries (**459-465**). This is fortunate for both patient and surgeon. The fusiform dilatation encroaches on the left side of the lumbar vertebral bodies causing backache. It extends forwards, pushing the intestines to each side so that it will eventually present as an easily seen swelling with a pulsation that expands. This can usually be readily differentiated from a transmitted non-expansile pulsation of the aorta in a nervous patient, which is a normal finding. The iliac vessels may also be aneurysmal, but often they do not need to be dealt with and can be left alone. This allows replacement of the aneurysm with a straight tube of dacron rather than a bifurcated one (**460-465**).

**459**

**460-465**  Sequential CT images through an aortic aneurysm starting below the level of the renal arteries.

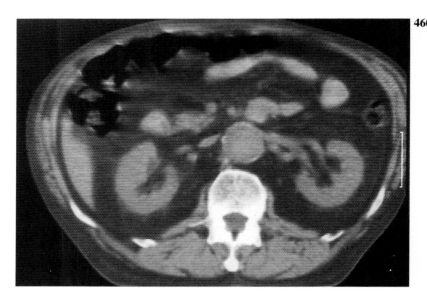

**460**

**460**  The aorta is mildly ectatic at 3.5 cm in diameter. The origin of the right renal artery can just be seen and a good length of the left renal vein and artery can be seen.

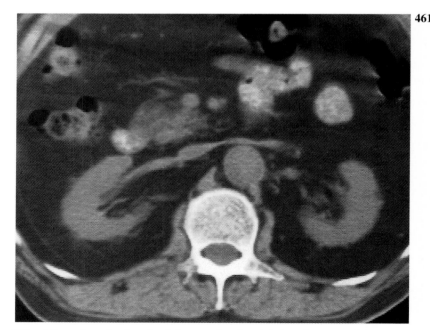

**461**

**459**  Typical anatomy of an aortic aneurysm showing the aorta crossed by the third part of the duodenum (D) and the left renal vein (R). A large lumbar vein which frequently enters the renal vein and encircles the left side of the aorta. The swelling will give a pulsatile expansion. The inferior mesenteric artery (M) usually comes out of the middle of the aneurysm. The relationship to the ureters (U) and vena cava (V) is close and important.

**461**  Viewed at the level of the renal veins joining the cava. The aorta measures 2·5cm across.

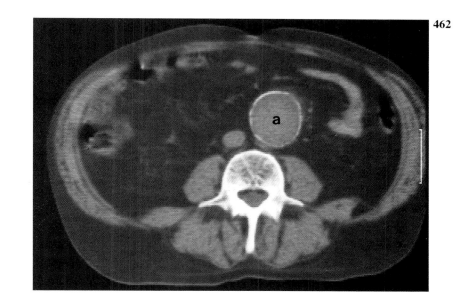

**462** An aneurysm (a; 5-cm diameter) is present below the level of the kidneys.

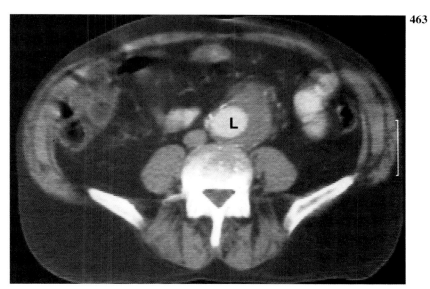

**463** The lumen (L) of the aneurysm is opacified by contrast medium. There is also extensive thrombus present; this is an invariable finding in a fusiform aortic aneurysm.

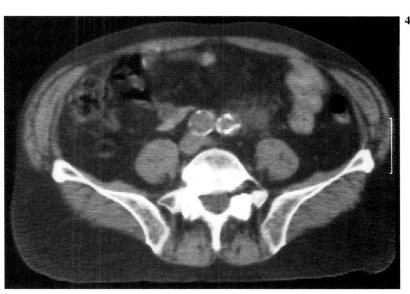

**464** The aneurysm has been traversed; normal calibre common iliac arteries.

At the operation, via a long incision, the caecum is mobilized and packed in a bag with the small bowel.

The inferior mesenteric artery is often occluded by the aneurysm, but whether or not this is so it must be ligated and divided. At the end of the operation the sigmoid colon is inspected to ensure its blood supply via the marginal vessel is adequate, which is usually the case. The ureters are identified and controlled with soft rubber slings.

The third part of the duodenum crossing the aorta is dissected off the vessel (465-469), revealing the left renal vein crossing the aorta to enter the vena cava. It is seldom necessary to divide this vein. A particularly troublesome vein, which should be deliberately ligated and divided, is the lumbar vein entering the renal vein, as otherwise it will probably be torn.

It is now usually possible to encircle the aorta, clamp it, and control the iliac vessels. When the aneurysm is opened the orifices of the segmental lumbal arteries will back bleed and are suture ligated. A dacron prosthesis is inserted and anastomosed above and below without resecting the aneurysm wall near the vena cava, which is another danger spot. It is a sobering thought that Astley Cooper was able to encircle the aorta by feel only, without damaging any other structure – but then he really did know his anatomy!

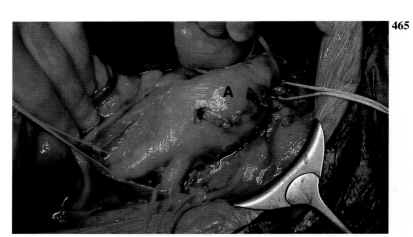

**465** Operative picture showing a large fusiform aneurysm (A) of the aorta which is also involving the common iliac vessels.

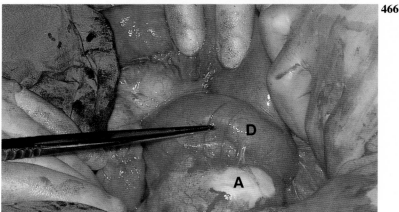

**466** Complication of an aneurysm in which the third part of the duodenum (D) has been eroded by the aneurysm (A).

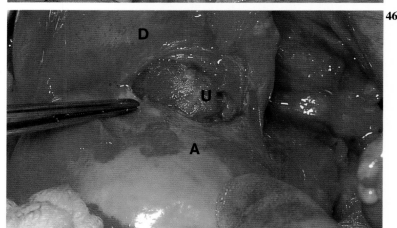

**467** When the blood inflow and outflow of the aneurysm was controlled, it was possible to remove the duodenum (D) from the aneurysm (A) and the ulceration between the aneurysm and the duodenum could be seen (U).

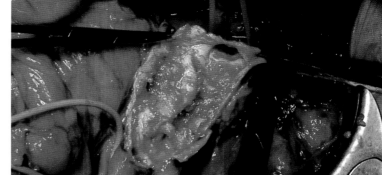

**468**  The inflow and outflow of the aneurysm has been clamped. The opened aneurysmal sacs can be seen from the inside.

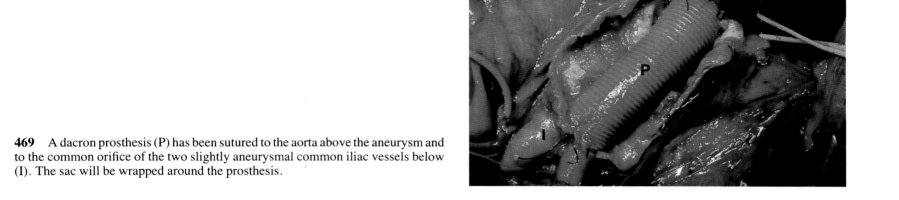

**469**  A dacron prosthesis (P) has been sutured to the aorta above the aneurysm and to the common orifice of the two slightly aneurysmal common iliac vessels below (I). The sac will be wrapped around the prosthesis.

# Index

**All figures refer to page numbers**